T0248199

FUTURE FORWARD

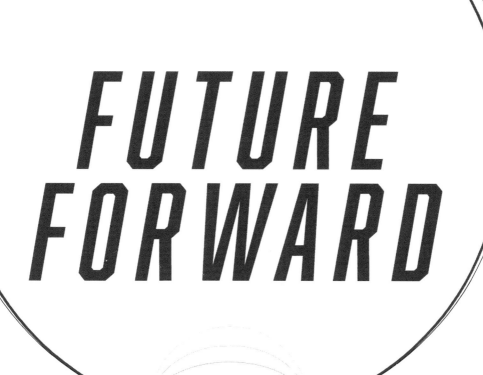

FUTURE FORWARD

LOOKING AT A POST-PANDEMIC WORLD

KEVIN CHEN

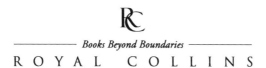

Books Beyond Boundaries

ROYAL COLLINS

FUTURE FORWARD
LOOKING AT A POST-PANDEMIC WORLD

KEVIN CHEN
Translated by Daniel McRyan

First published in 2023 by Royal Collins Publishing Group Inc.
Groupe Publication Royal Collins Inc.
550-555 boul. René-Lévesque O Montréal (Québec) H2Z1B1 Canada

ISBN: 978-1-4878-1033-7

To find out more about our publications, please visit www.royalcollins.com.

Foreword

PEOPLE HAVE GRADUALLY BECOME MUCH LESS FEARFUL OF THE COVID-19 pandemic thanks to effective treatments, vaccines, and herd immunity. Even if the virus cannot be eradicated, people have managed to master sufficient experience of coexisting with it for a long time in the past three years of fighting it.

On the one hand, the COVID-19 pandemic unexpectedly shattered the once linear, smooth, and predictable society. In a sense, it is a black swan event that has changed the course of human history. It has triggered a massive global crisis, dragging the world and each of us into a predicament not seen in decades.

The COVID-19 pandemic has infected hundreds of millions of people around the world and killed millions; it has dramatically impacted the political and economic patterns of the current times. During the COVID-19 pandemic, the global supply chain suffered a massive blow, further increasing the possibility of the global economy falling into a long-term recession. Then, this economic crisis has spread to politics, resulting in conflicts in geopolitical situations, social disintegration in some states, and an increase in the number of political earthquakes. The COVID-19 pandemic has exposed the deficiency of the existing global governance system of the U.N. and the W.H.O., which should have done a better job on this matter. Therefore, improving the level of international governance has become a significant and urgent task in the post-COVID years.

On the other hand, the COVID-19 pandemic has also presented a once-in-a-lifetime opportunity for change. As Winston Churchill once put it, a crisis is never to be wasted. History shows that choices made during emergencies can shape the global pattern for decades to come. World War II was not yet over when world leaders designed the postwar world at the Bretton Woods conference in July 1944. They had learned the lesson of the missed opportunity after World War I, so they understood that the focus must be shifted from ending the war to laying a new foundation, thus ushering in the "thirty golden years" of rapid global economic growth after the war.

Although the COVID-19 pandemic has led to a unique depression of global supply and demand, it has also accelerated the complex transformation of the worldwide economy. The heavy shackles were removed from the complex digital transformation, accelerating the formation of a long-term trend. And digitalization is covering more of people's life and work; the COVID-19 pandemic has pushed global information technology into a new stage of comprehensive penetration, accelerated innovation, and leading development. Also, it has sped up the arrival of the Fourth Industrial Revolution, deep integration of networking, informatization, and intelligentization. During the COVID-19 pandemic, a series of global risks have become increasingly prominent, including climate warming, the polarization between the rich and the poor, the crisis of antibiotic resistance, and ethical challenges, which forces all human beings to confront many global issues and collaborate to address them.

New worlds are emerging, but we have not yet outlined new blueprints. The truth is, the longer this pandemic goes on, the clearer it becomes that the virus is not a temporary disruption, and life will not return to what it was. The world before 2020 is history. And the optimistic times decades ago that were always open even though imperfect have vanished in this pandemic. At present, unexpected and rapid changes are still occurring in an endless stream. They merge, causing second, third, fourth, and more consequences, triggering chain reactions and unpredictable effects. From the perspective of the

COVID-19 pandemic alone, in addition to a remote end of it, with the intensification of environmental risks, people may face the next global pandemic any time soon.

Fatigue from the COVID-19 pandemic is not the best emotion to help people move on to new times. Getting used to it and making adjustments is what will genuinely help. When faced with various uncertain risks or opportunities in the future, we should at least have a basis. This book is based on this idea—it was written during the three years of the COVID-19 pandemic, covering a wide range of topics, spanning the fields of politics, economy, technology, ethics, and more. It discusses multiple hot issues of the COVID-19 pandemic and predicts the post-COVID world. It attempts to explain the possible changes in the future and to find specific clues in the uncertain drastic changes unseen in a century to establish a framework that can help us confirm our attitudes, lives, and ideals. And these simple confirmations are precisely the basis for an individual to find a position in an uncertain world.

Indeed, the only constant in this world is change itself. Uncertainty prevails in the objective world. Throughout human history, it has been normal for uncertain events to occur worldwide. History cannot prove it more. From the Black Death to the two world wars, these dramatic outbreaks have constantly changed the course of history. Therefore, uncertainty is even more fundamental than certainty. It is still too early to accurately describe how the post-COVID world will be reconstructed. However, this book hopes to provide rigorous and coherent content to help readers sort out the clues, re-understand the world amid the current and complex information, and make predictions about the development of related fields, society, and technology in the post-COVID years.

Contents

CONTENTS

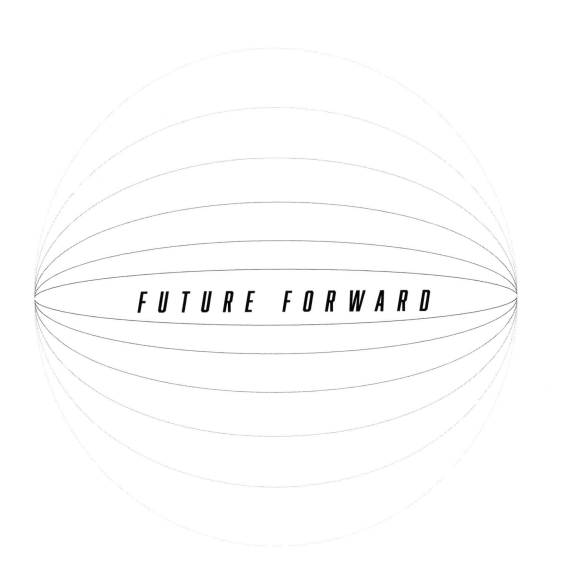

FUTURE FORWARD

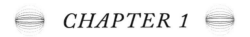

CHAPTER 1

Reconstruction of the Macroscopic World

SINCE THE OUTBREAK, THE COVID-19 PANDEMIC HAS BECOME THE MOST crucial variable affecting the global economy and international politics since the outbreak. It makes the international economic environment face "drastic changes unseen in a century." It is almost certain that the COVID-19 pandemic will, like all plagues in history, profoundly impact our social production and life. However, the effect of the COVID-19 pandemic on humanity will be far more significant than any other in history. Since World War II, it has had the most extensive, broadest, and most profound impact and challenges on human society. It will bring significant changes and tests to human life, social relations, trade relations, learning methods, and international political relations. Although the COVID-19 pandemic has resulted in a unique depression of supply and demand and geopolitical shocks, from a longer-term historical perspective, it has accelerated the complex transformation of global economic, political, and social governance.

Having exposed the shortcomings of globalization, the COVID-19 pandemic has changed the globalization and global trade system established in the past to varying degrees and will promote new and limited globalization. It has made the international political situation more volatile, led the world economy into a deep recession, intensified trade disputes, and escalated geopolitical tensions. Conflicts in political systems have begun to become apparent, and social conflicts within several countries have flared up, putting global politics and economics to the test. The pandemic has inflicted pain and incurred economic losses worldwide, further aggravating the K-type characteristics of the economic recovery and the polarization of different levels, categories, regions, and groups of people. The uncertainty of the pandemic also increases the possibility of religious conflicts, and it is inevitable to replace religious conflicts with civilized negotiation. The pandemic is testing the status and influence of the U.N. In post-COVID times, how the U.N. will play a leading role further and better coordinate all countries in the world to face the everyday challenges of humankind will become an outstanding problem that requires urgent solutions. The pandemic is no temporary social disruption but the beginning of a completely different macro world.

1.1 Future of the Pandemic—Risks, Options, and Paths

Whether it is a regional outbreak or a global spread, in the repeated mutation of the virus, the most frequently asked question is: Is it possible that the pandemic will end? It is more a complaint than a question. People are tired of wearing protective masks when they go out, tired of traveling under strict restrictions and the risk that a trip may end at any time, and tired of many less humanized treatments under pandemic prevention and control. Fatigue about the pandemic prevention and control is spreading.

Indeed, fatigue means nothing to the pandemic. The truth is, the longer this pandemic goes on, the clearer it gets that the virus is not a temporary disruption, and life will not return to what it was. The world before 2020 is history. And the optimistic times decades ago that were always open even though imperfect has vanished in this pandemic.

At present, unexpected and rapid changes are still occurring in an endless stream. They merge with each other, causing second, third, fourth, and more consequences and triggering chain reactions and unpredictable effects. From the perspective of the pandemic alone, in addition to a remote ending, with the intensification of environmental risks, people may soon face the next global pandemic at any time.

It is foreseeable that vaccines and specific drugs will become standard treatment methods against COVID-19. The virus will coexist with human society for a long time to come. Certainly, this is a helpless choice and compromise under globalization. Human society will have to deal with the virus similar to the common flu, meaning regular vaccinations or oral medication. Countries worldwide will eventually be forced to accept coexistence with the virus and resume international exchanges as long as the fatality rate is relatively controllable. For some time in the future, masks will be required for public travel activities.

But we have to notice the situation where the pandemic fails to be fundamentally controlled. As people continue to vaccinate and take oral medications, they are trying to fight against the virus utilizing immunization drugs. Judging from the current virus mutation, it is worse than any significant plague in history because the virus keeps evolving and mutating as it circulates the world. From Alpha, Beta, Gamma, and Delta, the mainstream variants in the first half of 2021, to the latest Omicron variant, it is clear that each mutation is taking place faster and becoming more infectious.

The generation of virus variants comes from mutations in the process of the virus's self-replication. The mutation comes from nature to humans and then goes from humans back to nature. There is also mutation after vaccine immunization. This cycle of mutation makes the virus unpredictable. To survive, the virus will continue replicating itself and mutate according to environmental changes. The more it reproduces, the more people infected, the wider the circulation, and the greater the probability and the number of mutations. Suppose human society fails to take decisive action to cut off the circulation of the virus as soon as possible, as the circulation continues. In that case, the mutated strain will make it easier for the virus to reproduce and spread faster, and the virus will develop strong resistance to vaccines and drugs during the mutation.

However, judging from the current global anti-pandemic situation, there are three different models, the social distancing model of solid control and dynamic zero clearing led by China, the free circulation model of the Western liberal and democratic countries led by the U.S., and the backward health protection measures in less developed regions such as Africa. Among them, mutation of the virus is most likely to occur in the third. Due to the lack of medical and sanitary conditions and popularized medical knowledge, the opportunities for people there to come into contact with nature and wild animals are much greater, which leads to the virus's circulation and mutation between humans, nature, and wild animals. This fundamentally allows it to mutate and break through. Then, with the flow of people, it is brought to the free West and spread to the whole world.

Vaccines and oral specific drugs cannot completely prevent the mutation of the virus because we cannot cut off the time and opportunity for it to mutate under a strongly controlled environment. On the contrary, every time humans apply upgraded vaccines and drugs, the virus gains a new chance for mutation, and it mutates to get stronger. Therefore, in the front of this great plague of humanity, if the whole world cannot cooperate to cut off the opportunity to spread and circulate the virus, it will not be easy to end. Human society must compromise and adapt to limited social distancing and mobility. As we coexist with the virus, we will continue to upgrade the antiviral drugs and be forced to accept irregular injections of vaccines and the administration of medicines.

But it may not be until after a generation of two that the sequela of these drugs shows. In other words, the potential risk to humans of these drugs developed via recombinant D.N.A. technology remains unknown. However, after a generation or two, new problems may break out. For example, sugar has changed the human diet. Over time, it has resulted in obesity, high blood pressure, and diabetes in human society, and they have become common diseases.

The virus is constantly mutating in its fight against humans. It may get stronger or weaker. But if we humans do not face up to ourselves and unite to fight the pandemic, the outcome will be that the virus will become stronger and stronger, and we will have to pay a painful price. One day, when we can no longer afford this price, we will wake up, start to change, and unite, except it may be too late. COVID-19 is the fascism of this century. If human beings do not unite and fight against it, it will be just an impossible dream for us to return to the free life before the pandemic. If the world does not act together to stop its spread, it will be difficult to eliminate it from the roots. In a few years, when we recall the good years of free breathing in the past, we will also think of time when some selfish humans indulged the spread, the mutation, and the upgrade of the virus.

The Endless COVID-19 Pandemic

Many few research reports have given enough evidence to analyze the future pandemic's possible direction. Among them, basic reproduction number (R0), vaccination efficacy, and antigenic drift are the most direct and scientific evidence.

R0 is the expected number of cases directly generated by one case. The estimated value of R0 is directly related to the spread of infection: when R0 is greater than 1, the disease will spread rapidly and become a pandemic, and if not prevented and controlled, it will grow exponentially; when R0 is equal to 1, the infection is local, controllable, and coexists with human beings for a long time; only when R0 is less than 1, will the disease gradually disappear by failing to spread.

The R0 of COVID-19 has also changed as its spread and study have deepened. At the beginning of the outbreak, researchers estimated that the R0 of COVID-19 was between 2 and 2.5, which means that in the absence of control measures, each infected case would infect about two people on average. However, researchers believe that the R0 of the mutated Delta variant is 5 or 6, 2–3 times that of the first R0, suggesting that the Delta variant is much more infectious where other conditions are the same.

Typically, the threshold for combined vaccine efficacy and herd immunity required for the disappearance of infection is calculated as $1-1/R0$. When R0=2, this threshold is only 50%. But when R0=5, to eradicate the virus, 80% of the people have to become immune to it. However, it is never easy to make 80% of the world's population immune, whether from vaccination efficacy or antigenic drift.

Although the COVID-19 vaccine is one of the best weapons for people to fight against the pandemic, as mutant strains continue to emerge, the virus seems to have broken through the vaccine's defense to a certain extent. Judging from the current global infection situation, some of the confirmed cases of the Delta variant have been vaccinated.

In early 2021, the La Jolla Institute of Immunology in California published a research report suggesting that people infected with COVID-19 can maintain the immunity for at least six months after recovery, and Public Health of England found that it was at least five months. The immunity obtained from the vaccine is basically the same as that obtained naturally from the infection, but their duration varies depending on each individual's constitution and health. It can last a long time or only a couple of months.

Regardless, it is inevitable that the protective efficacy of the vaccine is not 100%, and the effectiveness of antibodies declines over time. In fact, regarding the vaccines currently on the market, most of their immune efficacy can last for 6–12 months. Still, the duration varies depending on each individual's health and the types of vaccine.

Antigenic drift refers to the slight variation in antigens from a gene mutation. This kind of individual variation differs from the influenza virus's recombination. It does not produce new subtypes. It is a quantitative change without qualitative change. Mainly, it triggers a pandemic on a small or medium scale without having a significant impact on the virus. But if antigenic drift continues to accumulate, and the rate of accumulation keeps increasing, it will naturally sift out the viruses with greater infectivity.

Specifically, when COVID-19 first spread from animals to humans, it was not well adapted to the human body. In retrospect, the virus at the beginning was also the weakest since the outbreak. However, as it evolved, there have been rapid adaptive mutations in the S1 region of the spike protein, making it easier for COVID-19 to attack the human body.

Taking the Delta variant as an example, since it first appeared in India in late 2020, it has become the most widely spread strain in most regions of the world. It not only led to the rebound of the COVID-19 pandemic in Nepal and Southeast Asia but also spread wildly and dangerously in the United Kingdom and the U.S. It was found 60% more infectious than the highly contagious Alpha variant discovered in the United Kingdom at the end of 2020.

The Worst Variant

On November 26, 2021, the World Health Organization (WHO) sounded the alarm to the world after an emergency meeting about the new COVID-19 mutated strain B.1.1.529 in South Africa. It urged every country to stay vigilant and take counter-measures as the new variant spread worldwide. WHO deemed it a variant of concern (V.O.C.) and named it Omicron—the 15th letter of the Greek alphabet.

On November 26, 2021, South Africa reported 2,465 new confirmed cases on Thursday, twice as many as the day before and six times as many as two weeks ago. In only two weeks, the B.1.1.529 variant had replaced the Delta variant as the predominant variant among newly confirmed cases in South Africa, accounting for over 75% of the new total.

That night, WHO convened an emergency meeting on the new strain B.1.1.529 in South Africa. It skipped the usual intermediate stage and quickly identified it as a V.O.C.—the highest W.H.O. rating for variant severity.

According to whether the mutation of COVID-19 has enhanced infectivity and toxicity, the W.H.O. has classified the variants as variants of concern (V.O.C.), variants of interest (V.O.I.), and variants requiring further monitoring. Among them, V.O.C. is the one with the highest severity.

When I finished writing this book, Omicron had already been deemed the most lethal mutant strain of COVID-19 to date, and indeed, more variants will appear in the future. The number of mutations in Omicron and the importance of its mutation sites are far greater than those of the previously discovered V.O.C.s.

COVID-19 belongs to the same genus of β-coronavirus as SARS-CoV and MERS-CoV. It is the seventh type of coronavirus that infects humans and whose main structural proteins include the S protein (spike), E protein (envelope), M protein (transmembrane), and N protein (nucleocapsid). Among these four structural proteins, there are the most mutation sites on the S protein, meaning it is the most critical.

This is because the S protein is the critical protein for the infection of COVID-19 when it binds to the human body. The receptor-binding domain (RBD) on the S protein is also an important domain that binds to human cell receptors. And COVID-19 infects host cells by binding the RBD on the S protein to the ACE2 receptor on the host cells' surface, making it the target protein for most COVID vaccines to exert their protective efficacy.

As the name suggests, Omicron, the B.1.1.529 mutant strain, comes from the same B.1.1 lineage as Alpha (B.1.1.7). According to the science journal *Nature*, 32 mutations on its S protein are the highest number among all current variants. It is precisely twice that of the Delta variant. Meanwhile, Omicron shares multiple overlaps with the Delta and Alpha variants.

RBD is where the virus first contacts human cells. On the RBD of B.1.1.529, 10 mutations were found, making it the variant with the most RBD mutations, while the Delta variant, which has been raging worldwide, only has two. Mutations in the spike protein affect the virus's ability to infect cells and spread, making it difficult for immune cells to attack pathogens. Currently, most vaccines still rely on the spike protein to activate immune cells against COVID-19, meaning that Omicron may have far greater infectivity and broader spread than Delta.

In addition, there are H655Y, N679K, and P681H mutations near the Furin cleavage site of Omicron. The Furin cleavage site is located in the junction between the S1 subunit and the S2 subunit of the detected S protein of COVID-19. When the S1 and S2 subunits are cut from the junction via Furin, S2 can demonstrate how capable it is of helping the virus enter human lung cells, suggesting that the mutation of the restriction enzyme cutting site will significantly enhance the infectivity of the virus.

In addition, there is R203K/G204R mutation in the N protein of Omicron. According to previous studies published in *Cell*, the researchers have found that the R203K/G204R virus is highly adaptive through computational biology analysis. And through virus evolution analysis, it was found that R203K/G204R is related to the emergence of the highly infectious SARS-CoV-2 lineage B.1.1.7 (Alpha). In short, the 203K/204R mutation contributes to greater transmission and virulence of specific SARS-CoV-2 mutant strains.

Epidemiologist Eric Feigl-Ding cited epidemiologist J.P. Weiland's prediction that this variant may have an infection rate that exceeds 500% when compared to other variants. For the two most important epidemiological characteristics of Omicron, infectivity and immune escape, there is no specific data yet on B.1.1.529. We are still waiting for scientific identification and data publication.

Obviously, with developed modern medicine and informatization, despite the constant mutation of the virus, a human society shall not and cannot allow the pandemic to spread like wildfire. All the efforts people have made, whether it is restrictions on international travel or the research and development of COVID vaccines and specific drugs, are precisely to curb the spread of the pandemic and control the damage from it as much as possible. But unfortunately, the emerging new variants have posed a significant challenge to the existing governance system of human society. In the face of this pandemic, international organizations, including the W.H.O., have greatly doubted their organizational leadership and credibility. Therefore, if they do not reform, re-establish their professionalism and leadership, adapt to the new situation, and effectively improve their response and solution to major public health crises as soon as possible, it may be difficult for them to lead countries around the world to fight the pandemic.

Dynamic Zero Clearing and Coexistence with COVID-19

For now, the most likely future is us accepting COVID-19 as the new normal in our life. Indeed, when confronted with the objective reality of COVID-19 being the new normal, different countries have made other choices. There is "dynamic zero clearing" represented by China, and "coexistence with the virus" is also popular in Western countries.

Dynamic zero clearing is believed to be the most stringent policy in the world to prevent and control the pandemic. It immediately quarantines the source of infection and all close contacts and continues to adopt the approach of zero infection and zero transmission. The policy significantly distinguished China from other countries in the early stage of the pandemic prevention and control. According to the official reports of the *New York Times*, in March 2020, when the number of daily cases in other countries was tens of thousands or even hundreds of thousands, China contrived to control it within 100. This is not only a number but proof of the effectiveness of the "zero transmission policy.

Better epidemiological management has resulted in better economic performance. China was the only state to report a second-quarter gross domestic product (GDP) higher than that at the end of 2019 compared to the rest of the world. Vietnam, South Korea, and Hong Kong of China were close behind. China's success has prompted countries in the Asia-Pacific region, including Australia, New Zealand, and Singapore, to implement a similar policy, imposing lockdowns until the virus stopped spreading.

However, as new variants continue to emerge, especially the Delta variant, China's "dynamic zero clearing" policy has received more doubters. There are voices that the socioeconomic and public health costs brought by the Delta variant may be so high that they far exceed the benefits of prevention and control. But it should be noted that there are no winners in a society with a pandemic. It is about cutting losses. So far, China's pandemic policy has been a success.

Zhong Nanshan, an academician of the Chinese Academy of Engineering, concluded: "As China reopens to the world, a small outbreak of COVID-19 is inevitable, but with China's strong policy of monitoring the pandemic, including immediate identification of the patient zero, the chain of infection, the close contacts, and local testing of all residents, such an outbreak can be brought under control in a short period of time." And several small-scale local outbreaks have proved his words to be true.

The coexistence with the COVID-19 policy differs entirely from the dynamic zero clearing policy. It relies on vaccination to fight against COVID-19 while relaxing social distancing restrictions. Coexistence with the COVID-19 is the voluntary or forced choice of most countries. Both policies have clear pros and cons, but it is easy to tell which is better.

Taking the U.S. as an example, the Centers for Disease Control (C.D.C.) in the U.S. stipulates that patients should make an appointment for a COVID test according to their symptoms. If the result is positive, they need to self-quarantine at home for fourteen days or until they are asymptomatic and test themselves again after five to seven days of quarantine. When the result is negative, they are allowed to return to work. But when the patients self-quarantine, there is a greater risk of exposing their families, which leads to a massive increase in later costs.

A woman was self-quarantining at home for COVID-19 in Nebraska, and her husband had to stop working to care for their three preschool children, who could go to kindergarten every day without wearing masks because the children had not tested positive. This acceptance of the virus will eventually expose more families to being infected.

As of June 15, 2022, there were over 85 million confirmed cases and over one million deaths in the U.S. The U.K. had a higher fatality rate than the U.S. Some Asian countries like Singapore also joined the ranks to coexist with the virus, but, as expected, chaos took place.

Specifically, before the adoption of coexistence, the pandemic in Singapore was mainly in the dormitories for foreign laborers in early 2020. At the peak, about 1,000 cases were confirmed. There was little local transmission, and the virus basically subsided in August 2020. Under the outward-looking economic model, Singapore had a greater urge to open up than mainland China. With the high vaccination rate and abundant medical reserves, the country announced the new normal of coexistence with COVID-19 in late June 2021. At that time, regarding the level of vaccine protection, the Singaporean government optimistically expected that there would be at most hundreds of confirmed cases daily, and life would return to normal. However, the number of daily confirmed cases, hospitalized patients, I.C.U. patients, and deaths soared.

Since September 2021, the number of confirmed cases from community transmission has exceeded the previous peak of 1,000. It rapidly climbed to the level of 3,000 or 4,000. A new peak of over 5,300 daily confirmed cases was reached on October 23. It should be noted that this number was recorded after Singapore gave up tracking each patient. Generally, patients with mild symptoms were suggested to take medicines and quarantine themselves at home without reporting. In fact, the actual number of confirmed cases in the communities might be more alarming.

The number of hospitalized patients in general wards was a more accurate reflection of the pandemic. It has soared from less than 100 in July, exceeding 1,500 in October. Since September, the number of those infected with COVID-19 in the I.C.U.s has witnessed a gradual increase, too. Since mid-October, the number of COVID patients

13

in the I.C.U.s in Singapore has remained stable at around 70. There are about 60 more COVID patients in the I.C.U. due to their unstable conditions. In other words, they take up one-third of Singapore's 400 intensive care units.

Death tolls also surged in the past months. On September 30, the cumulative number of deaths in Singapore due to COVID-19 was only 95. The death toll has risen sharply in just over 40 days since October. As of November 13, 576 COVID patients have died. Considering the number of I.C.U. patients, the number of deaths is expected to increase for some time.

Statistics on the COVID-19 pandemic in Singapore as of November 13 show that there were 24,000 confirmed cases, of whom 72 were in I.C.U., 1,502 hospitalized, 23,000 under quarantine, and a total of 576 dead. It was an evident failure coexisting with COVID-19.

Life in the Pandemic-reshaped Society

Coexistence with COVID-19 means normalizing it as a common pandemic. And prevention and treatment are both indispensable links. From the perspective of prevention and control, vaccination and vaccine development remain the most effective ways; from the standpoint of treatment, the R&D of oral specific drugs is inevitable.

Regarding vaccination, although vaccines do not guarantee 100% protection, various vaccines are highly protective against mutant strains of COVID-19.

In mid-July 2021, *The New England Journal of Medicine* (N.E.J.M.) published the latest findings of Public Health England. The large-scale case-control and viral sequencing analysis of over 4,000 cases infected with the Delta variant show that the efficacy of two doses of the COVID-19 vaccine against symptomatic infection of the Delta variant is as high as 88.0%. Compared with the Alpha variant that had been widely prevalent in the U.K., the protection from the two doses was not significantly reduced.

We need to be reminded that vaccination needs to be complete. When there is one dose of the BNT162b2 vaccine, the preventive effect against symptomatic infection of the Delta variant (30.7%) was significantly lower than that of the Alpha variant (48.7%).

Similarly, where only one dose was administered, the effectiveness of preventing symptomatic infection of the Alpha and Delta variants was 48.7% and 30.0%, respectively. It is a wider gap.

Certainly, in the face of an entirely new virus, researchers have been studying several different types of vaccine candidates to maximize the chance of finding an effective solution. As the scientific community continues to tackle critical problems, as of July 2021, 20 intramuscular vaccines against COVID-19 have been approved for international use. At the same time, breakthroughs are being made in inhaled vaccines and oral vaccines. Hopefully, they can bring new options for vaccination.

For the treatment of COVID-19, people at first believed that it was a self-limiting disease. Like the SARS virus in 2002, there was no targeted drug to kill the virus, and recovery purely depends on people's immune systems. However, as the understanding of COVID-19 deepens, a series of specific medicines against it have begun to be seen.

There are two main ways to find specific drugs for COVID-19: biological macromolecular drugs based on antibodies and small molecular compound drugs that can inhibit virus invasion and replication. At present, the development of macromolecular biological medicines is progressing relatively faster, including monoclonal antibodies used as a single drug and the "antibody cocktail therapy." Antibody drugs have been approved for marketing or emergency use in the U.S., the U.K., Japan, and other countries to treat COVID-19.

Compared with macromolecular biological drugs, small molecular drugs have unique advantages in treating COVID-19. The targets of small molecular drugs can be distributed inside or outside the cells, while macromolecular biological drugs generally only act on the cell surface; most small molecular drugs can be administered orally, while macromolecular biological drugs can normally only be injected. The preparation of small molecule drugs is relatively simple and mature. Its yield is much higher than that of biological macromolecular medicines while the cost is lower, and the lower requirements for storage and transportation of small molecule drugs make it convenient to store and transport them.

However, the current small molecule biological drugs are mostly old drugs, such as hydroxychloroquine and remdesivir. The only new drug approved is Molnupiravir (MK-

4482, EIDD-2801), developed by the American multinational pharmaceutical company Merck & Co. On November 4, 2021, Molnupiravir was approved by the M.H.R.A. (Medicines and Healthcare Products Regulatory Agency) for treating adult patients with mild to moderate infection with COVID-19.

While Molnupiravir was approved, on November 5, 2021, Pfizer announced on its official website that compared with placebo, Paxlovid, its oral drug for COVID-19, reduced the risk of hospitalization or death by 89% in adult patients with mild to moderate infection with COVID-19 after the infected subjects took it within three days after having symptoms.

It is foreseeable that it is difficult for human society to return to the global free flow before the pandemic. Judging from the current situation, human society will be forced to accept the normalization of COVID-19 in the cycle of virus mutation and vaccine and drug upgrades. The combination of prevention and treatment through vaccines + drugs is of great significance in controlling the pandemic. This is undoubtedly the best strategy for the world to coexist with the virus in the future.

The Next Pandemic

Obviously, the COVID-19 pandemic has disrupted a once linear, predictable society, triggering a global crisis unprecedented in modern history. People expected that the vaccines would end the pandemic, but we now accept that the pandemic is still here despite the presence of vaccines. In addition, a risk must be noted from the pandemic's perspective that the COVID-19 pandemic may only be the beginning. In fact, as environmental risks intensify, there is the chance that the next pandemic may break out at any time.

On the one hand, more and more scientists are suggesting that it is precisely because human activities have destroyed biodiversity that new viruses such as COVID-19 emerged. Together, these researchers have launched a new research subject, Earth Health, which specializes in the delicate and complex relationship between human health and other biological species and the entire natural ecosystem. They have discovered that the destruction of biodiversity increases the number of pandemics.

As David Quammen put it in *Spillover: Animal Infections and the Next Pandemic,* there is a rich diversity of plants and animals and many unknown viruses in tropical rainforests and other wildlife habitats. When we invade these environments, cutting down trees, killing animals, or caging them for profits, we destroy their ecosystems and free viruses from their natural hosts. They need a new host, us humans.

In a letter to the U.S. Congress, 100 wildlife and environment protection organizations estimated that zoonoses (infectious diseases that have jumped from non-human animals to humans) have tripled over the past 50 years. Relatively, changes in land use have had the most negative impact on nature since 1970. Agriculture alone occupies more than 1/3 of the land area, becoming the economic activity that affects nature the most.

In addition, the researchers have found that the factors that promote agricultural development are related to over half of zoonoses. Human activities, such as agriculture, mining, logging, and tourism, invade natural ecosystems, and the boundaries between humans and animals have been broken, allowing infection to spread from animals to people.

The loss of an animal's natural habitat and the wildlife trade have a particularly significant impact on the emergence of wild diseases. For example, once bats and pangolins carrying COVID-19 are taken out of the natural environment and into cities, it is as if a distribution center for wildlife diseases is built in densely populated areas, dramatically increasing the possibility of zoonoses transmission.

On the other hand, global warming is inevitably melting glaciers in the North Pole and the South Pole. In 2020, large parts of Siberia suffered unseasonably high temperatures as the world was caught in the health and economic crises caused by the COVID-19 pandemic. This unusual heat has led to frequent wildfires, which burnt away the vegetation covering the permafrost, making it easier to thaw.

The consequences of this change are unknown but undoubtedly severe. In a report in *The Independent* in July 2020, Professor Jean Michel Claverie, a virologist at Aix-Marseille University in France, pointed out that viruses freed from glaciers and permafrost may be revived once they come into contact with a suitable host. Therefore, if humans are exposed to a previously frozen influenza virus, they can be infected, and a new pandemic may break out.

In August 2016, a 12-year-old boy died after contracting anthrax in the tundra of the Yamal Peninsula within the polar circle in Siberia, and at least 20 locals were hospitalized. One possible origin of this anthrax infection is that 75 years ago, a reindeer infected with the virus died, and its carcass was buried in the permafrost, which thawed in the heat of the summer of 2016, thus re-exposing the carcass and releasing anthrax into nearby water and soil. As a result, the virus entered the food chain, infected more than 2,000 reindeer grazing nearby, and eventually reached human beings.

Indeed, it requires academic research and more adequate confirmation of whether a once-lethal virus is still active after being frozen and released or its lethality is weakened. But under abnormal climate warming, environmental change has inevitably pushed us into a situation where we are at greater risk. The increase in uncertainty is closely related to climate change, but at present, people are far from vigilant.

Although human beings are accustomed to linearly picturing our future, we often ignore whether the world around us is working in a linear way, too. At present, COVID-19 keeps evolving in uncertainty, and where it will take human beings depends on their follow-up actions and attitudes. Half of the answer lies in the hands of the virus, while human beings hold the other half. The virus is uncontrollable, but human beings can make choices. The virus may not point straight to the answer but has already hinted at it.

It is foreseeable that COVID-19, with a limited mortality rate, is just a reminder from nature to the human society. It reminds us of two things: on the one hand, although we have turned the Earth into a global village through technology, where human beings seem to be closely connected, due to the conflicts of systems, concepts, cultures, and interests in human society, it is falling apart in the face of the virus, and there is a reluctance to unite to fight the pandemic because each party intends to maintain their own interests; on the other hand, with the advancement of science and technology, human beings are expanding their living space without limit, continuously occupying the natural space, which results in global warming, quicker melting of glaciers, and destruction of marine ecology. If we fail to exercise restrained self-discipline, the following more significant and lethal pandemic is around the corner.

I believe that the virus of the next pandemic will come from the mutation of marine viruses. On the one hand, the melting of glaciers has revived some unknown prehistoric viruses and released them into the ocean, and with the help of the marine ecosystem, they mutate. Next, they will enter the human society with marine organisms; on the other hand, we have damaged the marine ecology. Today, human beings are uncontrollably occupying the ocean space, and various pollutants are being recklessly discharged into the ocean, including Japan's nuclear waste, which will significantly destroy the marine ecology. When the habitat of unknown viruses and bacteria is destroyed, they will undoubtedly continue to mutate to survive. These mutated variants will take marine organisms as hosts, from whom they will further enter into human society.

The next more severe pandemic may not come from Earth. As exchanges between human society and space become frequent, on the one hand, some viruses and bacteria in human society may be taken into space, where they will mutate to survive. On the other hand, some space viruses and bacteria unknown to us might enter the spacecraft we make and come to the Earth and mutate. Therefore, as human beings' exploration, exploitation, and competition in space continue to intensify, the mutated viruses from space will become a hidden hazard to which we must stay alert. Today, in the name of scientific and technological advancement, human society is selfishly and uncontrollably occupying Earth and space. And we are deeply concerned about the consequences.

1.2 From Globalization to Limited Globalization

The COVID-19 pandemic that ravaged the world in 2020 changed the economy and society and significantly impacted the pace of globalization. It directly blocked the regular exchanges of the international economies and made people rethink the impact of globalization on the economies and social security of various countries. The pandemic has led nations to reflect on the pros and cons of globalization, including how to ensure the safety of their own industry and supply chains. However, this does not mean that globalization is going backward. Instead, it is seeking new development and building a new development model. In a way, the new globalization will be limited globalization.

Total Globalization

Globalization refers to the global economic integration characterized by international trade and investment. It is the inevitable result of economic and social development. Since the Age of Discovery, the trend toward globalization has begun to surface. With the development of transportation and communication technologies, the Earth has gradually shrunken into a village, a common home for all people. One key indicator to judge the degree of global economic integration is the proportion of international trade in Gross Domestic Product (G.D.P.). According to this indicator, globalization of the world in modern times can be divided into three stages:

First was the golden age of international trade from 1846 to 1914. In 1842, global merchandise exports accounted for less than 4% of global G.D.P. By 1913, and the proportion had reached 14%; the value of world trade soared from 640 million pounds in 1851 to 7.84 billion pounds in 1913. However, the sudden outbreak of World War I rained on the fiery globalization. Even if there was a short economic recovery after World War I, the Great Depression happened, de-globalization followed (marked by sharply higher tariffs in various countries), and eventually World War II broke out.

The second stage was from the end of World War II to the end of the 1970s, during which international trade and investment within the Western coalition led by the U.S. took a giant leap. In contrast, trade and investment cooperation coexisted within the Eastern alliance led by the Soviet Union. This was the second peak of global economic integration. In the late 1960s, international merchandise trade accounted for about 20% of global G.D.P. After the energy crisis in the 1970s, this proportion changed constantly, but until the early 1990s, it remained at around 30%. It is worth mentioning that the globalization in this period was not true globalization but a globalization of coalition.

The third stage is from the 1980s to the present. China, the former Soviet Union, and Eastern European countries have one after another undergone economic transformation. They have joined the economic system dominated by Western powers and formed a true global economic integration, characterized by the formation of global industrial chains and value chains. Since the early 1990s, the share of global merchandise trade has skyrocketed, reaching 40% in 2000 and almost 52% in 2008. International merchandise trade is linking more countries, and the degree of economic integration continues to deepen through trade. The annual growth in global trade volume reached 3% from 2000 to 2006 and climbed to 6.5% in the year before the financial crisis.

After the outbreak of the financial crisis in 2008, global trade and economic growth shrank sharply. The share of international merchandise trade in global G.D.P. dropped by 10%. After the world-shaking financial crisis, trade intensity bounced back, but the percentage of trade in economic growth did not. Before it, trade was growing at roughly twice the rate of global G.D.P., and now the two grow at the same rate. Therefore, there is concern about whether international trade has peaked. While absolute trade volume may keep expanding as the world's population continues to grow, in terms of relative trade volume, perhaps it has indeed peaked.

It has been proven that the global division of labor is by far the most efficient production method, which can maximize the potential of worldwide demand and optimize the allocation of the Earth's resources. Human society's transformation from manual production mode to mass machine-based industrial mode promotes the expansion of the social division of labor and commodity exchange, the further integration of the global market, and the increasingly close economic ties between countries. Everything develops under its objective laws. However, this wave of globalization has gradually led to more negative outcomes. The pandemic has forced us humans to calm down and think more deeply about the current models and future direction.

Disadvantages of Globalization

At present, the adverse effects of globalization have triggered widespread concern and attracted global attention.

First, there is the emergence of global problems, which are problems that have a significant impact on and pose a severe threat to the survival and development of the entire human race on a worldwide scale. In fact, since the publication of the Club of

Rome's 1972 research report *Limits of Growth*, various global problems in the relationship between man and nature have attracted great attention around the world, including environmental pollution, ecological imbalance, population explosion, food shortages, energy shortages, resource depletion, etc.

Indeed, the problem of the ecological environment is no unique problem in contemporary times. Having existed in the form of clues and signs as early as modern times, it has undergone a long-term evolution with the development of a modern industrial technology civilization. However, with the development of globalization, especially with the expansion of industrialization to every corner of the Earth since World War II and the application of various modern technological means on a global scale, the damage to the ecological environment in contemporary times has at last broken through the tolerance limits of nature. Therefore, a general and cumulative result, namely, a global environmental crisis, broke out. In short, contemporary globalization has continuously intensified and eventually escalated the problem of the ecological environment that has existed for ages into a global problem. And these global problems challenge the familiar and comfortable lifestyle of those with vested interests.

The second negative impact is the global power transfer. From the 19th century, during which European powers vied for overseas colonies, to World War II, Europe was widely considered the center of power in the world. During this period, it was both the base of the contenders and the region of strategic contention. As colonialism continued to develop, the strategic fight among European powers began to spread to areas outside Europe, but Europe remained the main area vied for by European powers. From World War II to the end of the Cold War, the U.S. and the Soviet Union were the two strongest powers in the world and the two most critical strategic competitors in the international system. The Soviet Union was located in Europe. Meanwhile, the focus of competition between the U.S. and the Soviet Union during this period was also in Europe. Therefore, it remained the world's power center during the Cold War.

However, since the 1980s, on the one hand, significant countries in the third world have begun to rise. Japan played the game of capitalism more skillfully than Europe and the U.S, and China and the "seven tigers" of Southeast Asia, free from the influence of Western liberalism, started their own path to wealth. In particular, the characteristics of

China's comprehensive national strength forced the U.S. to take China as the biggest rival in the 21st century, which marks the shift of its most significant strategic competitors from Europe to East Asia.

On the other hand, the West fails to compete with their increased productivity and shrinking workforce. Under the impact of the financial crisis since 2008, both Europe and the U.S. have suffered a decline to a certain extent. And the decline of Europe has made it less influential than East Asia, which immediately replaced it as a component of the world center. The relative decline of the entirety of Europe, including Russia, is one of the reasons for the shift of the world's power center. In addition, no country in Europe has the potential to become a global superpower, while China, located in East Asia, does.

Although China is confronted with problems of people's well-being, anti-corruption, the legal system, and the gap between the rich and the poor, the country's leaders are clearly aware of them and are trying to solve them. Despite the U.S.'s rising absolute strength, the power gap between China and the U.S. is shrinking because China is growing faster than the U.S.

Third, globalization is deviating from the original objective. Initially, globalization aimed to create an economic and trade community of free countries and societies. However, in actual practice, the social, political, and legal structures of many late-developing countries lack liberalization, which gives state capitalism the chance to intervene in the process of globalization, which leads to an unequal competition for a free economy and intensifies the unbalanced development of the world. Globalization has caused an unprecedented polarization between the rich and the poor in different regions, countries, and classes.

Statistics show that the wealthiest 1% of the world's population owns more wealth than the rest of the population combined. The wealth of the relatively poor half of the world's population has grown by only 1% since the 21st century. In the U.S. and many other developed countries, incomes for the middle-class have stagnated over the past 40 years. Unbalanced global development has led to drastic changes and even transformations in the international social and political trends of thought. Nationalism, populism, protectionism, and extremism have prevailed. There has been chaos in the international economic and political order, with "trade wars," "withdrawals from associations," and "withdrawal from treaties." And global security threats like terrorism are on the rise, too.

Over the past three decades, countries enjoying globalization's benefits have ignored the emerging problems and risks. Among them, the most significant problem in the U.S. is that in the 30 years before the pandemic, it allocated too much energy to play the role of the policeman of the world and neglected the optimized solutions to the increasingly severe domestic problems such as racial conflicts, social innovation, and social governance. Although former U.S. President Donald J. Trump's strategy may seem crude, it is not a bad strategy for restructuring and revitalizing the country.

The U.S., which is deeply caught up in the pandemic, with the hegemony of the U.S. dollar, has overissued U.S. dollars, accumulated massive debt, made excessive global interventions, and hollowed out industries. Capital has deviated from real investment to virtual investment, industrial workers have been unemployed, large arms dealers have kidnapped the U.S. economy, the military expenditure has been too high, and there has been insufficient investment in people's well-being, serious aging of infrastructure, a vast gap between the rich and the poor, bitter social divisions, noticeable political differences, and ineffective control of guns and drugs, etc. All these are accelerating the disappearance of the advantages of American society. And the pandemic has completely exposed these disadvantages. On the one hand, it has sped up the outbreak of internal problems in the U.S.; on the other, it has brought the old model of globalization led by the U.S. to an end.

Reconstruct the Globalization Pattern

Although COVID-19 is not the first global pandemic, it has undoubtedly highlighted the objective existence of global problems and significantly strengthened people's cognition and reflection. Obviously, the COVID-19 pandemic will not return human society to the old patterns of independent governance and sovereign supremacy before globalization. Changes and advancements in science and technology, economic life, and knowledge make it impossible for human beings to stay out of globalization. No country can develop independently without it. It is an inevitable future that will enter a new stage of globalization.

The advancement of science and technology decreases the manufacturing industry's sensitivity to the factors of production, making it possible for limited globalization to occur. In the past, globalization prompted factories to migrate to regions and countries with low production costs. However, as science and technology continue to advance, many factories have realized production with fewer or zero workers. Therefore, scale production is no longer the most critical variable that the industrial chains consider, which also makes it possible to establish diversified industrial chains in the future in the three continents (Asia, Europe, and America). As regional organizations grow, limited globalization will present the characteristics of "blocking."

For example, the Regional Comprehensive Economic Partnership (R.C.E.P.) is a free trade zone mechanism with the largest population, the most significant development potential, and the most diverse membership structure globally. It signifies the common will of all countries in a region. As one of the largest international associations, the R.C.E.P. has 15 member states, including ten ASEAN countries and China, Japan, South Korea, Australia, and New Zealand, who accommodate 30% of the world's population, hold nearly 30% of the global G.D.P., and over 27% of global trade volume, surpassing those of Trans-Pacific Partnership Agreement.

R.C.E.P. integrates and optimizes the five "ASEAN+" countries to form a unified regional system. This cooperative and transparent institutional environment makes it possible for multinational companies to allocate resources according to their comparative advantages and to reconstruct and optimize the division of labor and industrial chains in the region, which helps reduce operating costs and enhance their overall competitiveness in the region. Moreover, the fifteen member states of R.C.E.P. are highly complementary. There are countries with cutting-edge technologies such as Japan and South Korea, countries with intensive labor such as Vietnam and Cambodia, and countries with abundant resources like Australia. In theory, if R.C.E.P. members can closely cooperate, they can form a relatively complete industrial chain and supply chains and shelter all member states against external storms, like the broken global supply chain on a large scale caused by the COVID-19 pandemic.

The form of "blocking" appeared decades ago, such as with the European Union, ASEAN, African Union, etc. However, in the post-COVID-19 times, when global integration is struggling, it is most likely for "blocking" to evolve. Due to the regional correlation within the block, there is a greater interest correlation. In addition to the greater cultural commonality and closer traditions in the same region, whether tangible or intangible, material or non-material, it is easier to solve problems and cooperate within the block. Blocks for a while will become a developmental trend in the future, and the connection between blocks will form a global relationship.

In addition, from whatever point of view, the practice of this global fight against the pandemic helps deepen the understanding that countries worldwide must unite to address global problems. On the one hand, people are made to see the objective reality of the imbalance in various countries' responses. Besides developing countries with little capability to control COVID-19 from going wild and who require the support of developed countries, even the world's largest powers like the U.S. cannot handle it alone. On the other hand, people are made aware that if the meaning of solidarity and mutual assistance is not understood from a global perspective, as long as COVID-19 remains uncontrolled in any country, it will keep threatening other countries. It is practically necessary to unite and cooperate.

Totally different from the way of understanding and solving problems in international relations, since the outbreak of the COVID-19 pandemic, there has been no consideration of winners and losers. No country is alone in this fight. The urgency and importance of building a community with a shared future have become more evident in the responses to this global public health crisis. The repair of the international governance system and the multilateral system still matters. This requires humankind to face up to the future development tendency, to the role of multiple forces in global governance, the sequence in the restoration of the international governance system, and how the tools are combined to repair it. Only when united can the international community overcome the pandemic.

The COVID-19 pandemic will not end globalization but will only rewrite part of its framework. It continues to go on in post-COVID times, but it is bound to be reconstructed, and the reconstruction will inevitably bring about a new pattern of globalization. The current Sino-U.S. relations have added some variables to this reconstruction. The U.S. has more cutting-edge technologies and R&D talents, while China holds a vast market and, more importantly, a more complete manufacturing chain.

It has been predicted that the future globalization will be a process of collision, conflict, exchange, and integration of the old world system led by the U.S. and the new system of a more open, inclusive, and cooperative 'community of shared futures' built by the emerging power China. It is expected to take place within the next thirty years. As two major powers with global influence, Sino-U.S. cooperation plays a pivotal role in the sustainable stability and prosperity of human society. The collision and conflict between the old and new systems will be intense in the upcoming first decade. If the U.S. does not rigorously implement the one-China principle and continues to intervene in Taiwan affairs, a hot war over the Taiwan issue will likely break out. The "community with a shared future" advocated by China is not a disintegration and reconstruction of the old world system, but an upgrade and optimization of the current globalization system. In the face of global problems, such as climate change, anti-COVID actions, and international trade, China and the U.S. will still hold irregular leaders' meetings and discussions. Both countries will figure out a way to cooperate despite their disagreements and find a new balance until a new tacit understanding is formed.

If Sino-U.S. tension can be alleviated, and if they can join hands, the technological advantages of the U.S. and China's complete industrial chain will promote the development of the world economy to the greatest extent. However, if they continue to be in the current state of absolute confrontation, if the U.S. continues to uphold a Cold War mentality, to stay hostile toward the Communist Party of China and the Chinese government, to implement the anti-China and China-excluded policies, and to suppress Chinese enterprises and high-tech progress, there will be a significant adverse impact on the economic development of the U.S. itself. Global economic prosperity and human development will suffer.

The confrontation between China and the U.S. will affect the development of the world economy to a certain extent and increase the cost of living in other countries to a certain extent. Although the U.S. is still trying to charm some allies to "besiege" China with its leader's charisma, this strategy is objectively not the optimal solution, and Western countries should objectively face up to China's current values, problems, and strengths. Instead, the strategy of cooperation and fair competition with China is the best solution to a globalization strategy in post-COVID times.

Obviously, the ongoing pandemic has made countries reassess and think about the impact of globalization. They have become unconsciously concerned about their supply chain vulnerability and economic dependence at the level of national economic security. It is foreseeable that no matter what Sino-U.S. relations become, countries worldwide cannot afford to wait. If Sino-U.S. relations remain in the current conflict and confrontation situation, the world polarization pattern will speed up. After the pandemic, a new and limited globalization model will appear faster.

1.3 Greater International Political and Economic Uncertainty

The stability of the global macro environment is inseparable from the two cornerstones of international political cooperation and global economic exchanges.

International political cooperation refers to the partnership between sovereign states. It is the transfer of jurisdiction over economic affairs from the national level to the international level. Because of the anarchy in the international community, the orderly conduct of economic activities can only be ensured by establishing rules, sanctions, and contingencies. For example, the World Trade Organization (W.T.O.) regulates trade, the International Monetary Fund (I.M.F.) oversees financial activity, and the Basel Committee on Banking Supervision supervises the banking system. The global economic exchange reflects the economic connection in the spatial dimension. It is the further subdivision of the division of labor in the industrial chain, the expansion of the distance between the production market and the consumer market, and the extension of economic activities from the regional to the global level.

The global macro environment will be at its best when both elements are present. However, in recent years, western populism led by the U.S. has risen, unilateralism and protectionism have warmed up, and geopolitical games have been more frequent. Under these circumstances, the extreme climate and the impact of the COVID-19 pandemic in 2020 have added more volatility to the global political situation. Compared with before, the global economic pie has again shrunk sharply, the economic development has been unbalanced, the deep structural problems in the West have intensified, and some governments and politicians that have been dumping the blame are making global politics and economy more unstable. The irrational Sino-U.S. confrontation started by the U.S. will only lead to more internal friction that means little to all countries involved.

Turbulent World Politics and Economy

The economic basis determines the superstructure. In fact, the reasons behind the occurrence of geopolitical conflicts, social disintegration in some countries, and the increase in the number of political earthquakes on a global scale are the long-term economic downturn, unbalanced development, and structural problems. It plagues all the governments worldwide in that how far the prosperity sustained by the continuous over-issue of currency can go. The higher prices of commodities because of over-issued currency will have a far-reaching impact on the lives and consumption of everyone.

In 2008, the U.S. financial crisis and the subsequent European debt crisis forced central banks in the West to conduct bold, unconventional currency experiments. While the experiments avoided another great depression and boosted the capital markets, the actual economy stagnated, and public and enterprise debt grew at an alarming rate. In 2020, twelve years passed since the two crises. However, Europe and the U.S. have not only failed to resolve the deep structural problems, but their economic development has moved toward more significant imbalance and inequality. Also, the long-term slump and imbalance of the economy have nourished populism. The governments or politicians in some western economies are accustomed to shifting domestic conflicts. They adopt protectionism and unilateralism, causing geopolitical tensions.

The sudden outbreak of the COVID-19 pandemic in 2020 has brought the global economy to a standstill and has loosened the international economic linkages. The division of labor in the industrial chain is intended to use comparative advantages and save production costs, but the pandemic has exposed the adverse effects of this practice. The global layout of the production line determines that as long as one of the links breaks, the entire chain will suffer. It inevitably accelerates companies' active withdrawal of their global industrial layout to build a closed and complete value chain system in the region. The ebb of international economic exchanges is salt in the wound of an unstable macro environment.

Under this circumstance, European and American central banks have followed suit, deepening unconventional monetary policies again, relying on market paths, and piling up financial assets. Compared with before, the global economic pie has again shrunk sharply, the economic development has been unbalanced, the deep structural problems in the West have intensified, and some governments and politicians that have been dumping the blame are making the global politics and economy more unstable.

Meanwhile, the conflict between the China-led socialist system and the U.S.-led western liberal democratic system is escalating because China is growing stronger. Thanks to China's continuous development, reform, and opening-up, and with the release of domestic demand potential, the Chinese economy is expected to maintain a medium-to-high growth rate. The long-term economic improvement lays a foundation for the stability of the capital market. In addition, China continues to deepen the reform and opening up of the capital market. Although it has become the world's second-largest economy and the second-largest bond market and stock market, there is still a considerable amount of real assets that have not been financialized in China. Therefore, compared with the development of the real economy, with the accelerated internationalization of the Chinese RMB and the continuous advancement of asset financialization (the newly established Beijing Stock Exchange being the most direct expression of intention), there is enormous space for China's future capital market development.

Undoubtedly, as the two largest economies in the world, only when China and the U.S. cooperate can they unite with the rest of the world. However, during the pandemic, the U.S. seemed to spend the most energy on non-constructive behaviors on the international stage, such as stigmatizing the virus, attacking the W.H.O., and demanding compensation from China. Behind these behaviors lies the underlying logic of its global actions: after seeing China as a strategic competitor, cooperation has changed to confrontation.

At present, the world is at the time after both the financial crisis and the COVID-19 pandemic. The western economies have been sluggish for a long time, internal structural problems and conflicts have intensified, and geopolitical tension has risen. Inevitably, weakening the global economic foundation will exacerbate the overall political instability. At the same time, the U.S. relied on the international monetary system of the U.S. dollar, established by itself, and the asset-pricing power it held to issue currency without restraint, which triggered global inflation during the pandemic. This move has obviously reduced the hegemonic influence of the U.S. dollar to a certain extent and prompted more countries to consider the RMB settlement system instead.

While the U.S. relies on the hegemony of the U.S. dollar to issue currency without restraint, the Chinese RMB shows restraint. It maintains considerable firmness and stability. It is foreseeable that "the internationalization of the RMB" will start from the cooperation of countries involved in the Belt-and-Road Initiative (B.R.I.) and spread slowly. It is expected that after 2035, it will become one of the world's mainstream currencies of settlement, weakening the current hegemonic advantage of the U.S. dollar.

Along with a series of conflicts in the global economy and the steady development of the Chinese economy, the heart of the global economy has shifted, and the heart of international political influence has also moved eastward. After the pandemic, this trend will be more visible, and the global political and economic situation will be more volatile.

Break the Deadlock

In the face of international political and economic turmoil, breaking the deadlock is necessary. For the short term, prevention and control are the prerequisites for the restart of economic activities. The first and foremost is still effective pandemic prevention, blocking the spread of the pandemic and accelerating the research and development of vaccines or specific drugs. As the most economical and effective means to prevent and control infection, the successful development of vaccines is the key to the ultimate control of the COVID-19 pandemic. As many COVID-19 vaccines have been approved for conditional marketing or emergency use around the world, the global vaccination for COVID-19 has picked up, leading to a continuous drop in the number of new confirmed cases in a single day globally. However, at the national level, because of the gap in vaccine acquisition, transportation, and inoculation, it is difficult to synchronize the vaccination in high-income and low-income countries.

In these times of globalization, no one will be safe unless everyone is. With the steady inoculation of the COVID-19 vaccine, the number of COVID-19 cases worldwide has shrunk significantly. While the economies of various countries gradually recover and open up, as an RNA virus, COVID-19 is constantly mutating. Every variant carries stronger transmissibility from the Alpha B.1.1.7 to Beta B.1.351, Gamma P.1 and Delta B.1.617.2. The prevention and control of the pandemic remain a challenging task.

Economically, in the short term, countries should also implement precise and effective fiscal and monetary policy support to alleviate the massive impact of the pandemic on the real economy, to reduce the bankruptcy of small-, medium-, and micro-enterprises, and to avoid interruption of the industrial and supply chains, and the short-term impacts become long-term. In China, as per sampled business data, the operating income of small- and medium-sized enterprises (S.M.E.) in the first quarter of 2020 was less than 50% in the same period in 2019, and more than 80% of SMEs faced cash flow problems. Among them, SMEs in education, catering, accommodation, sports and entertainment, and manufacturing suffered the most significant blows from the pandemic.

The turnover of SMEs in the education industry in February and March 2020 was only 10.2% and 11.8% in the same period in 2019. Such percentages of SMEs in the accommodation and catering industries were only 12.8% and 23.5%, those of SMEs in the sports and entertainment industries fell below 30%, and those of SMEs in the manufacturing industry were less than 40%. Surviving the crisis has become an unavoidable problem for SMEs in post-COVID times.

In the medium and long term, countries need to eliminate their dependence on short-term stimulus policies gradually and, under specific rules, maximize factor mobility to improve economic efficiency, increase employment and income, and release demand. And this requires reform and global free trade. Reform will be inevitably painful. From the perspective of the various economies since the outbreak of the financial crisis in America and the debt crisis in Europe, there are many obstacles to reform. The western authorities have the intention, but not the determination and vigorous action.

As for global free trade, the benefits are apparent, such as lowered trade barriers, and rule-based free trade competition is conducive to promoting the free flow of factors. This makes global investment and trade thrive, increasing employment, and reducing poverty and uneven development. And then, there will be an effective division of labor and co-operation among countries, and the improvement of total factor productivity will release potential global demand. This boosts sustainable economic growth, earns broader public support for reform, gradually resolves deep-seated conflicts in the countries' coordinated development, optimizes their national balance sheets, and stabilizes the global political situation.

At present, some developed economies still hold ideological discrimination. They maintain their advantages by restricting the development of other countries. However, the actual results show that their economic downturn not only triggers strong counter-measures and confrontations but continues to escalate geopolitical tensions.

Whether it is China, the U.S., or any other country in the world, working together to control the pandemic has always been the best choice, and humanity should not blindly go towards self-destruction. Therefore, at the beginning of April 2020, hundreds of scholars from China and the U.S. urged countries to stop accusing each other and cooperate. How to conduct international cooperation in the future dramatically tests the vision, self-discipline, and determination of political leaders of various countries. To a large extent, the post-COVID world depends on the choices made today by the politicians in multiple countries, which will determine the stability of the global macro environment.

Judging from the current situation, the West, led by the U.S., has failed to take effective measures to control the pandemic. The rotational mutation of vaccines and viruses will further escalate the harmfulness. To truly safeguard the world's interests, the U.S. should exert its world leadership and influence to control completely, cut off, and destroy the transmission chain of the virus within a quarter. Giving the world a normal order as soon as possible is how America should show its leadership and values.

And the more countries will see through the selfish strategy of the U.S., which puts itself first. It will have to slowly give up its global leadership, narrow its strategy, and retreat to North America step by step. It is impossible to expect the U.S. to lead the world in the fight against the pandemic and eradicate COVID-19. Without a miracle, COVID-19 will never disappear overnight but will continue to spread, upgrade, and mutate. Humanity will only truly wake up if it has to keep paying the price of significant public health crises. And long gone is the U.S. that once shouted in World War II that it would become the arsenal of democratic countries, fight for the justice of all mankind, and ultimately defeat fascism.

1.4 Economic Nightmare

The COVID-19 pandemic has caused pain and economic losses around the world. However, the policies aimed at controlling it have also raised the asset prices, benefiting the richest the most. In most countries, the gap between the rich and the poor is widening. An estimated 5.2 million people became millionaires last year, and the number of those with assets worth at least US$ 50 million rose by nearly a quarter.

Every major human crisis accelerates the widening gap between the rich and the poor. On the one hand, since the stock market crash in March 2020, the U.S. index and the Shanghai Composite Index have made new peaks after a V-shaped rebound. The capital market reflects investors' confidence in the future. On the other hand, the stubbornly high unemployment rate and the weak job market suggest that economic recovery still has a long way to go.

As the gap between the rich and the poor widens, its negative effects have become a great concern. If extreme economic imbalances are not alleviated, more violent social unrest or global conflict will break out. Like all great plagues in history, which also resulted in some "disruptive innovations," this pandemic has also offered the world an opportunity to think about coexistence.

Origin and Causes of the Wealth Gap

The gap between the rich and the poor is a social law. There is a vast polarization between the rich and the poor worldwide, and since the 1980s, the distribution of income and wealth in most countries has deteriorated.

Globally, from 1980 to 2019, the income of the top 1% climbed from 17.10% of the total global income to 19.34%, an increase of 2.24%; the income of the bottom 30% experienced only a rise of 0.57 %, and the income of the middle 40% fell from 41.86% to 39.29%.

Taking the U.S. as an example, according to the data from the WID, in 1939, the income of the top 10% accounted for 47.8% of the total income in the U.S., and that of the bottom 50% was 14%. World War 2 narrowed the income gap. By 1945, the incomes of the top 10% and the bottom 50% accounted for 35.6% and 19.7% of the total, respectively. After that, the percentages have remained at this level until the 1980s.

After 1980, the gap between the rich and the poor quickly widened. By 2018, the incomes of the top 10% and the bottom 50% accounted for 46.8% and 12.7% of the total in the U.S., respectively. The gap was 34 %, a level comparable to that of 1939. And the U.S. income Gini index has been above the warning line of 0.40 for the past 20 years.

The same is happening to other developed countries. The income of the top 10% in the E.U. ascended from 29.61% of the total in 1980 to 35.15% in 2019, an increase of 5.54%, while that of the bottom 50% decreased from 22.56% to 20.08%. Since 1980, the incomes of the top 10% in Germany and France have both been around 30% of their total; in Russia, since the disintegration of the Soviet Union in 1991, the rich have quickly accumulated the most wealth. The income of the top 10% has risen from around 20% of the total to 50%.

Meanwhile, the income gap in developing countries is also widening, and the Gini index has long been above the warning line. Taking China as an example, its reform and opening-up have significantly boosted the economy. Still, at the same time, it has widened the gap between the rich and the poor. In the early days of reform and opening up, the top 10% earned the same amount of wealth as the bottom 50%. But 40 years later, the gap between the two groups has widened by 38%. In 2017, the wealthiest 20% of Chinese held 45.8% of the total social wealth, close to the number of the U.S. (46.9%) over the same period, surpassing Germany, France, and the U.K. (39.7%, 40.9%, 40.6% respectively), while the poorest 20% owned only 4.2%.

Fundamentally, the factor reward that directly affects the primary distribution and the relevant factors that lead to the polarization between the rich and the poor through redistribution is to be blamed.

Regarding the factor reward that affects the primary distribution, on the one hand, the general laws of economic development and industrial transformation directly expand capital accumulation and aggravate the polarization between the rich and the poor. The relative surplus of labor and the relative scarcity of capital results in a higher marginal rate of return on capital. Under the premise of private ownership of the means of production, capital owners will enjoy more benefits than labor providers, thus polarization.

On the other hand, factors such as technological progress and globalization have changed the wage income of workers with different skills and widened the gap between the rich and the poor. Technological progress casts an asymmetric impact on workers, meaning highly-skilled workers receive higher wages, creating an income gap. Under global economic integration, this labor market split has been further amplified.

Regarding the relevant factors that lead to the gap between the rich and the poor through redistribution, the increasingly severe gap between the rich and the poor is related to the abundant possession of financial resources of the rich and the long-term low effective interest rate. Regarding the former factor, if the factor reward in the primary distribution affects the gap between the rich and the poor, the financial resources advocated in the market economy significantly aggravate social wealth inequality.

The core function of finance is to promote the efficient allocation of resources, whose scarcity will lead to the flow of market resources to the most efficient sectors to improve efficiency further. However, due to the existence of information asymmetry and moral hazards in the market, when financial institutions deal with various types of investors to save human and material costs and improve the efficiency, they will always choose to serve companies or individuals that have consistently performed well and reject potential or disadvantaged demanders.

In addition, the "resource combination effect" encourages more wealthy people with a broad horizon and sufficient capital to choose stocks, funds, and foreign currency for portfolio investment, to obtain higher returns at lower risks. For example, for the rich in the U.S., the top 5% of wealthiest families hold 85% of the stocks, while the low-income families possess few financial assets and almost zero stock. Therefore, the rich obtain higher investment returns under this asset portfolio, becoming even wealthier, while the poor become the opposite.

Long-term low effective interest rates further make it easier for the rich to possess more financial resources. Taking the U.S. 10-year treasury bond interest rate as an example, in 1919, the interest rate level of treasury bonds was around 5%, and during World War II (1939-1945), it dropped to 2%; after the war, it soared until peaking at 14% in the early 1980s; since the mid-1980s, it continued to fall, and by the end of 2019 it was around 2.2%.

In this case, the rich can maintain and increase their wealth through diversified property transfer channels and diversified investments. In contrast, the poor face higher loan constraints due to their low wealth level and less access to financial resources. This implicit "inflation tax" has undoubtedly redistributed social wealth and widened the gap between the rich and the poor.

The COVID-19 Pandemic Widens the Gap

Every major human crisis accelerates the widening gap between the rich and the poor. In the COVID-19 pandemic, the gap between the rich and the poor has widened again globally through emergency economic policies, higher asset prices, and the asymmetric impact of the pandemic. Consequently, a K-shaped recovery pattern was formed.

With the cliff-like economic downturn, high unemployment rate, and low commodity prices that come with the COVID-19 pandemic, central banks of various countries restarted and created a series of monetary policy measures to deal with the crisis. The monetary policy means that they used can be classified into three categories: interest rate adjustment, open market trading, and credit easing.

Interest rate adjustment was the first policy the central banks adopted. After the outbreak of the pandemic, the Federal Reserve Bank of the U.S. and the Bank of England lowered their benchmark interest rates twice in March 2020. Among them, the Federal Reserve lowered the federal benchmark interest rate by 50 basis points (bps, where one basis point is equal to 1/100th of 1%) and 100 bp on March 3 and 16, respectively, maintaining the target federal interest rate range at 0–0.25%, which has remained unchanged since then. Bank of England lowered its benchmark interest rate by 50 bps and 15 bps on March 11 and 19, respectively, to a historic low of 0.1%. Before the outbreak of the pandemic in the Eurozone and Japan, the benchmark interest rate levels were already at or below zero, so the central banks did not adjust them again.

Secondly, central banks around the world conducted an open market operation. For example, the asset class that the Federal Reserve has bought more of is treasury bonds and mortgage-backed securities (M.B.S.). It first announced purchases of $700 billion, including $500 billion in treasury bonds and $200 billion in M.B.S., and then promised there would be no cap on asset purchases. Except for March and April, monthly asset purchases remained at $120 billion.

The expanded asset purchase plan released by the European Central Bank (E.C.B.) consists of two parts. One is the regular asset purchase program, whose new monthly bond purchase scale is 140 billion euros (of which 120 billion will be implemented until the end of the year 2020). The other is the Pandemic Emergency Purchase Program (P.E.P.P.), including purchasing private and public sector bonds. The initially announced purchase scale was 750 billion euros and expanded to 1.85 trillion euros in December. The purchase program was extended to March 2022, and the reinvestment of the principal recovered from P.E.P.P. was prolonged to the end of 2023.

The assets purchased by the Bank of Japan included treasury bonds, ETF, J-REITs, corporate bonds, and commercial paper. Among them, there was no cap on the purchase scale of Treasury bonds; the annual purchase target of ETF was six trillion yen, with a total scale of twelve trillion yen; that of J-REITs was 180 billion yen; the total purchase amount of corporate bonds and commercial paper was twenty trillion yen (the ceiling quota for corporate bonds and commercial paper per issuer was raised to 500 billion yen and 300 billion yen, respectively), and the purchase program was implemented until September 2021.

Lastly, central banks around the world have also performed credit easing. After the outbreak of COVID-19, the Federal Reserve Bank of the U.S. restarted and created many credit support facilities that directly targeted entities such as residents, enterprises, and governments. There are three main categories. The first is the facility used by the U.S. Department of the Treasury to inject capital from the foreign exchange stabilization fund; the second is the Primary Dealer Credit Facility (P.D.C.F.) and the Paycheck Protection Program Leading Facility (P.P.P.L.F.), neither of which do require financial subsidies; the third is the C.A.R.E.S. (Coronavirus Aid, Relief, and Economic Security) Act special appropriation.

The E.C.B.'s credit-easing facilities mainly include the T.L.T.R.O.s (Targeted Long-term Refinancing Operations) III and the P.E.L.T.R.O.s (Pandemic Emergency Long-term Refinancing Operations) in response to the pandemic. The former is a targeted loan issued to families (excluding housing mortgages) and non-financial enterprises (excluding the public sectors). The loan interest rate was adjusted twice during the year to a range between –1% and –0.5%, which is lower than the E.C.B.'s refinancing benchmark interest rate. The proportion of loans obtained by banks from the E.C.B. through this monetary policy tool was raised to 55% of the loan stock in 2019, and the cumulative loan volume in 2021 reached 1.65 trillion euros. The latter mainly provides liquidity support for the Eurozone's financial system. In 2021, it operated seven times, injecting a total of 26.7 billion euros of liquidity into the market. The execution time of the two facilities was extended to the end of June 2022.

But whether it is interest rate cuts, open market operation, or credit easing, the most direct outcome is the continued expansion of the central banks' balance sheet and the continued easing of global liquidity. Inevitably, they will lead to inflation in post-COVID or post-crisis times. The prices of various assets will be more expensive due to the over-issued currency.

For the wealthy, most of their currencies will be allocated in the form of all types of assets, and the result must be that their personal assets will expand as asset prices rise. A Credit Suisse report shows that global families' total wealth rose by about $28.7 trillion in 2020 as central banks flooded financial markets with cheap capital, raising asset prices.

The rise of equity and housing real estate valuations has boosted the total family net asset (including real estate minus debt) to about $418.3 trillion. That equates to a 4.1% growth when a fixed exchange rate is calculated. It was slightly lower than the annual average of the past 20 years, even as the global economy struggles to cope with the impact of the COVID-19 health crisis and corresponding lockdowns.

The Credit Suisse report estimates that there were 56.1 million millionaires worldwide at the end of 2020, an increase of 5.2 million from the previous year. And about one-third of the new millionaires are from the U.S. The changes in family wealth stand in unprecedented contrast to what is happening in the broader economy.

However, this is clearly a disaster for low-income and middle-income groups because it is difficult for their incomes to increase significantly. Still, the commodities they consume have become more expensive because of the increased asset prices. In addition, they do not have sufficient money to diversify their asset allocation. As a result, they have to suffer from the pressure and challenge of inflation.

In addition, due to the enormous financial losses from the economic recession caused by the pandemic, some groups such as less educated employees and low-paid employees are suffering a more significant blow. One way to assess the resilience of these groups after the pandemic hit them is to look at their job characteristics, such as the ability to work remotely and the necessity of jobs and interpersonal communication. An IMF report, having summarized the differences in the importance of these job characteristics across U.S. industries, found that industries that require more human interaction. For example, the leisure and hospitality industries tend to have higher unemployment rates, and sectors that have suffered severe damage tend to have a relatively lower job necessity. The reason is that the ability to work remotely is highly correlated with education levels, and employees with less education are more vulnerable to the impact of the pandemic, which further widens the income gap.

The pandemic might also widen the gap between developed and developing economies, which have weaker healthcare systems or find it difficult to cope with domestic outbreaks. As a result, strict lockdowns and social distancing in developing economies will likely last for a long time, leading to mass unemployment. Some emerging Asian countries have inadequate social security systems, and there are the most significant gaps in current financial support schemes to secure jobs, leaving low-skilled workers more vulnerable. In addition, the virus's continued spread has slowed the international population flow, and the income gap between developed and emerging economies may widen more due to a decline in tourism and fewer immigrant workers.

The Global Problem of the Gap Between the Rich and the Poor

The acceleration of the widening gap between the rich and the poor is evolving into a global problem whose negative effects are concerning.

The most direct impact of the accelerating widening gap between the rich and the poor is the hindrance to economic growth. In the short term, it leads to sluggish consumption and insufficient effective demand, further restricting economic growth. Naturally, the rich have a lower marginal propensity to consume than the poor. As the gap between the rich and poor widens, the socially weighted average marginal propensity to consume declines, resulting in insufficient consumer demand.

First, in the long run, the widening gap between the rich and the poor will lead to weak innovation momentum, lower average education levels, and lower total factor productivity, thereby impeding economic growth. On the one hand, technological innovation requires support from market demand. With the widening gap between them, the social income structure goes polarized, and the middle-income group has been dramatically shrunk, weakening the support for technological innovation to a certain extent. On the other hand, the widening gap narrows the living space of S.M.E.s and entrepreneurs and directly affects the development prospects of innovative entities.

Second, the widening gap between the rich and the poor has a self-reinforcing negative feedback effect. For a relatively poor individual, the most critical constraints restricting consumption are income and wealth, so a higher salary encourages more consumption. Because most of the consumption demand has been met for a reasonably wealthy individual, only a small fraction of the income raised will be used for consumption while the rest becomes savings.

As a result, a low effective interest rate leads to a widening gap between the rich and the poor. As the consumption of the rich increases relatively little, and the poor have no income to support consumption, the overall consumption demand of the society will go down, and the lack of demand might further force the government to loosen monetary policies. For example, in response to the declining consumption after the 2008 financial crisis, the U.S. lowered the interest rate to 0.25%. The decline in the nominal interest rate further accelerated the expansion of the wealth of the rich, forming a self-reinforcing gap between the rich and the poor. For this feedback mechanism, a widening gap between the rich and the poor could have a kind of "multiplier effect" on the economy.

Finally, the widening gap between the rich and the poor also triggers socio-political problems. There are more signs that it has intensified the conflict among all social classes, which is marked by the prevalence of populism, the stronger tide of anti-globalization, and the rise of political parties with extreme ideologies, which are threats to international and domestic politics and economy. The rich are changing while the polarization is not. The accelerated widening of the gap between the rich and the poor is becoming a global problem. If extreme economic imbalances are not alleviated, more violent social unrest or global conflict might break out. As Confucius said more than 2,000 years ago: "Those who rule worry more about uneven distribution than little distribution." This should enlighten us in the post-COVID times.

1.5 Nonnegligible Possibility of Religious Conflict

Since the 1970s, a series of major incidents related to political Islam has drawn the attention of the political and academic circles to it. Especially after the Iranian Revolution, the political Islamists of Sudan came to power, the Algerian elections, the 911 terrorist attack, the Arab upheaval, and so on, in the context of counter-terrorism, the relationship between the West and political Islam has become a key factor affecting international relations.

Although the relationship between the West and Political Islam has entered a new period, due to the fundamental conflict of interests and power between them and the cultural, religious, and ideological clashes, the tension between the two parties will last for a long time. Though the lockdown during the pandemic is decreasing the global fertility rate, the Islamic population may suffer a smaller blow because of their religious concept that the more, the merrier. In the future, as the foreign Islamic population grows, it is more likely for religious and political conflicts to take place.

Origin of Religious Conflict

Historically, the conflict rooted in the cultural background of Islamic civilization and Western Christian civilization constitutes the main thread of the relationship between the Islamic world and the West. When Islam was founded in the seventh century A.D., Christianity had matured. However, Islam, which advocated the expansion of jihad and the establishment of the Islamic world order, expanded outwardly at an alarming scale and speed, arousing a strong shock and extreme hatred in Western Christian society. As a result, the opposition and conflict between the Christian West and the Islamic world fully unfolded.

In fact, Islam had the upper hand in several early conflicts. As Arnold Toynbee, a famous British historian, put it, the first encounter between Christianity and Islam occurred when Western society was still a baby. At that time, Islam was a unique religion in the glorious age of the Arabs, who had just conquered and reunited the territories of the ancient civilizations of the Middle East, and planned to expand that empire into a world state. In that conflict, Muslims almost occupied half the territory of the West and nearly became world masters. In the clash between Christianity and Islam, the fall of territories, the destruction of Christian holy places, and the failure of the Crusade left indelible scars on the hearts of Western Christians, who were constantly trying to defeat Islam.

The Renaissance and the religious reforms in the sixteenth century made Western Christian society take a step toward modernization. Especially after the bourgeois revolution in the 17th and 18th centuries, the advanced political system, brilliant material civilization, and the accumulation of massive primitive capital in the West woke the superiority complex of the Christian society. Once again, the Islamic world, as an old enemy, has become the subject of its conquest. At this time, the Muslim world was no longer facing a belligerent Christianity during the Crusades, but missionaries, educators, business people, cannons, fleets, science, and technology. It suffered defeat and humiliation from the West, where there were new cultures and a new order of life. Since the 18th century, the confrontation and conflict of conquest and anti-conquest, preaching and anti-preaching between the West and Islam have been in full swing.

After World War II, with the rise of the national liberation movement of the Islamic countries in the Middle East, Arab nationalism emerged in the political arena of the Middle East, and those nationalism factors constituted the central theme of the confrontation between Islamic countries and the West. Some politicians who pursued Islamic reformism once tried to absorb the modern West's advanced political and economic systems and humanistic ideals to modernize the Islamic countries. However, years of reforms failed to save a fading Islam. Instead, the social crisis caused by modernization and the West's support for Zionism once again aroused the intense disgust of the Muslims against the West. Therefore, since the 1970s, both the Islamic revival movement that has spread across the Islamic world and the rapidly rising Islamic fundamentalism organizations have taken opposing the West and purifying Islam as their primary goals. Consequently, the conflict between the two cultures was ignited again.

Fundamentalism raises anger into a denunciation and criticism of Westernization and modernization. Because secularization does not agree with Islamic tradition, the fact that it is imposed on Islam leads to total social alienation and endless troubles. Westernization means colonization, and the Western model will only make Islamic countries vassals of the West. Secularized education will disorientate Islamic education, and the consequences of secularization will trigger a political crisis. The rule of secularized pro-Western political elites will make the regime lose public support. This fundamentalism not only proposes to negate Westernization but contains the proposition of seeking introversion from the perspective of value orientation—Islamic civilization is a self-sufficient ideological system that can respond to the challenges of the times and achieve future revival with its abundant cultural resources.

The Iranian Revolution that broke out in 1979 fundamentally shook the strategic presence of the U.S. in the Middle East. The Ayatollah Ruhollah Khomeini made anti-Westernism one of the primary goals of Iran's foreign policy, which deeply disturbed and panicked the U.S. The Gulf War in the 1990s appeared to be a fight only between the U.S. and Iraq. Still, the strengthened strategy of the U.S. in the Middle East also triggered anxiety in most Islamic countries, and anti-Western sentiment continued to rise. In recent years, the military and economic sanctions imposed by the West on Iran, Libya, Iraq, and Afghanistan have further fueled the hatred of the Muslims against the U.S.

After the 9/11 terrorist attacks, some Christian right-wing conservative forces in the U.S. government believed that the terrorist attacks launched by al-Qaeda actually reflected the discontentment of the Islamic world against the Western Christian world headed by the U.S. They thought that the conflict between the U.S. and the Islamic world embodied by the 9/11 terrorist attacks was actually a continuation of the conflict between the Western Christian world and the Islamic world over a thousand years ago. Therefore, they strongly appealed to the U.S. and the Western Christian world that it represents to fight back.

For example, on September 16, not long after the 9/11 terrorist attacks, U.S. President George W. Bush publicly used the term "crusade" in a press conference to express his understanding of the nature of the terrorist attack and his anger toward Islamic extremism. It was an attempt to ignite the patriotic enthusiasm of most Americans, mainly Christians, and their dissatisfaction with Islamic extremism. Although the White House spokesman denied the "crusade" in his subsequent speech, saying that President Bush only had a slip of the tongue, it is an unavoidable fact that behind the aggressive foreign policy in the name of combating global terrorism in the U.S. lies indeed a religious complexity between traditional Christianity and Islamism.

In retrospect of the history of the relationship between the Islamic world and the West, the conflict constitutes the central theme of their relationship. It was partially a cultural conflict. Moreover, under the nation-state system, the main body of the conflict is the state, while the cause of the conflict is the fight for interests and power. The damage that Western countries have inflicted on the fundamental interests of the Islamic world is the root cause of political Islam's opposition to them.

In addition, if the conflict between Western countries and Political Islam involves cultural, religious, and ideological factors, the two sides' shared idea of antagonism formed in the long history is the root cause of their conflict. And it has led them to identify each other as enemies under the reciprocal mechanism. And the rise of Political Islam not only poses a real threat to the hegemony of the U.S. in the Middle East but challenges the West as an anti-Western ideology.

According to its historical experience of secularization, the West holds a "conservative, backward, and radical" impression of Political Islam that engages in politics in the name of religion. Under the catalysis of Islamic radicalism, "Islamic threat" and "Islamophobia" spread wildly in the West. For example, it is a common belief in the West that Islam is a rigid religion that cannot keep up with the times; that it shares no common values with other faiths; that it is a barbaric, outdated, and irrational religion that is inferior to the West; that it supports terrorism; and that it is a political ideology that advocates violence.

Although the relationship between the West and Political Islam has entered a new period, due to the fundamental conflict of interests and power between them and the cultural, religious, and ideological clashes, the tension between the two parties will last for a long time.

The Trend of Muslimization

As the Muslim population expands in Europe, the trend of Muslimization in Europe is growing stronger. At the end of the 19th century, when capitalism transitioned to imperialism, many European countries accelerated their colonial expansion in Africa, Southeast Asia, and other places. During this period, as a means to consolidate colonial rule, they were delighted to invite and finance the upper classes of the colonial countries under their jurisdiction, especially the young generation, to study and work in Europe to cultivate their cultural closeness and political identification to their colonizers. Many of them chose to settle in Europe, and most were Muslims.

A larger wave of Muslim immigration happened after the end of World War II. To solve the labor shortage problem and boost economic recovery, European countries began to encourage and accept immigrants, thus attracting a large number of Muslim laborers from the Middle East. Since the 1970s, more Muslims have come to Europe to work and join their families. Meanwhile, as turbulence continued in Syria, Afghanistan, Libya, and other places in recent years, the number of war and political refugees entering Europe reached a new peak.

At present, Muslim immigration keeps going. In addition, the Muslim immigrants who entered Europe in the early years have already given birth to the second and third generations. The proportion of European Muslims in the total European population continues to expand. In 2016, the Muslim population in Europe reached 25.8 million, accounting for about 5% of the total European population as the biggest minority in Europe. In terms of country distribution, France and Germany have the largest Muslim populations, 5.7 million (8.8%) and 5 million (6.1%) respectively, and 25% of the young French citizens under the age of 25 are Muslims.

It is worth mentioning that the lockdown because of the COVID-19 pandemic in 2020 will affect the global fertility rate in the long run, and there will be unstoppable differences. From the growth trend, for countries with high welfare, such as those in Europe, the lockdown and the pandemic's blow on the economy and society will shrink the fertility rate of local residents. In the meantime, the impact of a low fertility rate on negative population growth is delayed and hidden, and it is a long-term process of continuous accumulation and gradual manifestation rather than an "immediate result." However, because of religious consciousness, Islam advocates having more babies, meaning a smaller blow from the pandemic on fertility. Moreover, compared with non-Muslims, European Muslims have a younger demographic structure and are more willing to have children. It is foreseeable that with the increasing number of foreign Islamic populations, the trend of Muslimization in Europe will grow stronger. After 2035, there will be wider Muslimization and Turkification in Germany, France, the U.K., or even the entire European Union.

The increase in the Muslim population and the increasingly explicit Islamic cultural characteristics may complement the mainstream values of European countries and destroy the traditional European cultural attributes, thereby shaking the dominant social position of locals. In terms of religious culture, most European Muslims strictly abide by Islamic teachings, upholding Allah's will with a weakened status of humans. This collides violently with the mainstream European individual rights and freedom, rationality and equality, and adherence to secularization. Recently, it has been hotly disputed in Europe whether women can wear hooded robes in public, whether schools are obliged to provide halal meals, and whether the government should limit the rapid expansion of mosques. If in the future, because of population decline European nations have to increase the number of immigrants due to population decline, and most of the new immigrants are Muslims, it is perhaps inevitable for conflicts to break out between European countries and Muslims.

Replace Religious Conflict with Dialogue Among Civilizations

Undoubtedly, in the current globalization, it is of great significance for different nations, different states, and the entire world to recognize the basic development tendency of world civilization and adopt a correct and effective cultural strategy. Contrary to the idea that the clash among civilizations is inevitable, more and more people have realized that only by replacing the clashes with dialogues among civilizations can humanity join hands to build a better world.

Anwar Ibrahim, former Deputy Prime Minister of the Federal Government of Malaysia, made a convincing argument on the need for "dialogue among civilizations" in a speech he gave at a U.S. university in October 1994. He stressed the importance of communication between Asian civilizations and Western civilizations. He believed that as globalization accelerates, people from different regions and cultural backgrounds will have more frequent exchanges. Simultaneously, as a reaction to globalization, people will have a deeper awareness of cultural identity and civilizational differences. Therefore, the most outstanding significance of the dialogue among civilizations is their better mutual understanding through sincere and friendly exchanges, the elimination of prejudice and misunderstandings through communication, and the foundation laid for their extensive cooperation.

Anwar emphasized that to achieve positive results in the dialogue between Asian and Western civilizations, both need to bury the hatchet and see each other with a developmental and forward-looking perspective. Therefore, the Islamic world should overcome its grudge over the Crusades and colonial rule towards the West. At the same time, the West should set aside pride and prejudice towards the East and the Islamic world and see Islamic civilization from a new perspective.

The dialogue among civilizations is both necessary and urgent. Thanks to the active intervention and promotion of the U.N., more and more countries will gradually recognize such dialogues. In September 1998, former Iranian President Mohammad Khatami suggested that U.N. member states pass a resolution to designate 2001, the beginning of the 21st century, as the U.N. Year of Dialogue among Civilizations. This proposal reflected the mainstream public opinion worldwide and was approved at the General Assembly in November 1998.

To implement the spirit of the U.N. General Assembly resolution, with the joint efforts of the countries concerned, the First International Symposium on Dialogue among Asian Civilizations was held in Tehran, the capital of Iran, in February 2001. After that, a declaration on the basic principles and significant insights of the dialogue among civilizations was made. It emphasized that all human cultures have rich cultural heritages and have made important contributions to world civilization, that equal, friendly, and sincere dialogue should be made among and within each society to enhance mutual understanding, and that based on seeking common ground, we shall share the common values of humankind, and actively and effectively respond to the threats and challenges mankind encounters in the fields of peace, security, ecological protection, and poverty elimination; and that governments, regions, and international organizations, especially the U.N., which shoulder a vital mission, should take practical actions to encourage, promote and support dialogue, exchanges and communication among various civilizations.

Historically and practically, the conflict between the Islamic world and the West is deeply cultural. As an extraordinary soft power, culture has always played a specific role in the tussle between the two sides. Once the conflict becomes cultural, both parties will identify and judge the international conflict according to their measured values and humanistic standards and seek a cultural definition that conforms to their value identification for their political actions and goals. Therefore, the sublimation and internalization of the fight for interests and power into cultural pursuits are culturally legitimate. But such conflict is not entirely irresolvable—only by seeking common ground while allowing differences to exist can human civilization evolve to a higher level.

1.6 Sino-U.S. Relations Determine the Course of Global Politics and Economy

Sino-U.S. relations are one of the world's most complex and critical bilateral relations. After the Cold War, the U.S. became the only superpower in the world. But today, the collective rise of emerging countries represented by China has had an objective impact on the global hegemony of the U.S. China's global leadership continues to grow stronger, while that of the U.S. is declining.

On February 28, 2019, Gallup Inc., a famous American polling company, released a report on the public opinion in 2018 about the global leadership of the world powers, including the U.S., China, Germany, and Russia. People from 133 countries around the world participated in the survey. The results showed that Germany ranked first with a 40% support rate, which was the first time it had such a low rate in ten years; China came second with 34%, the highest rate in ten years; the U.S. was the third, at 31%, 1% higher than the previous year; Russia was the last, slightly under 30%, almost equal to that of the U.S. The report suggests that China's leadership has gained a greater advantage in the competition for world power.

Since the reform and opening up, China has witnessed a soaring development for over 40 years, becoming the second-largest economy after the U.S. It is increasingly apparent that it is catching up with the U.S. and is likely to surpass it. It is a common opinion in the U.S. that China is the most likely challenger to its hegemony. The international community also believes that China and the U.S. have the relationship of a challenger country and a hegemonic country in the international system.

The present world is a globalized, integrated, and diversified world, as well as a complex world where comprehensive national strength is paramount, technology is the most potent weapon, and great powers compete. By the middle of this century, China is expected to surpass the U.S. and become the world's largest economy in terms of total economic output. However, it is still behind the U.S. in comprehensive national strength. In this context, Sino-U.S. relations will be essential in determining the course of global politics and economy.

Sixty Years of Sino-U.S. Relations

From 1949 to the present, Sino-U.S. relations have gone through two thirty-year periods and entered the third. In the first thirty years of the Cold War and the Korean War, China and the U.S. were in two rival camps and brutal wars between them during the Cold War.

First, there was the Korean War. When it broke out in June 1950, the U.S. extended the battlefield to the banks of the Yalu River on the northeastern border of China, and from time to time, it sent planes into the territory in northeast China to provoke China. China was forced to fight back. In October 1958, it deployed a volunteer army to fight side by side with the Korean People's Army, and 2.4 million volunteer soldiers entered the D.P.R.K. and dauntlessly fought bloody battles with the troops of sixteen countries led by the U.S. At last, the U.S. had to sign an armistice agreement in 1953.

The second was the Vietnam War. From 1964 to 1973, the U.S. successively deployed over 540,000 soldiers in the Vietnam War. After over 58,000 soldiers died and more than 100,000 were wounded, it retreated from Vietnam. During the Vietnam War, China sent over 300,000 soldiers to Vietnam. Still, China did not directly participate in military operations like the Korean War but helped Vietnam train troops, support logistics, and draw battle plans.

The hostilities between China and the U.S. eased in 1972. In 1972, then-President Richard M. Nixon visited China and normalized Sino-U.S. relations. It was a diplomatic move with far-reaching influence. After establishing diplomatic relations between China and the U.S. and Deng Xiaoping's visit to the U.S. in 1979, their cooperation ended the cold war in East Asia.

The second thirty years is when China started the reform and opening up and continued to blend into the global economy. On January 1, 1979, China and the U.S. established diplomatic relations, and both countries entered a period of win-win cooperation. In January 1979, Deng Xiaoping visited the U.S., laying a solid foundation for their honeymoon period. After consultations, the two countries co-issued the *Three Communiqués* in 1982. Taking this as an opportunity, their relationship entered what was later widely known as the honeymoon period, during which they maintained an excellent interaction based on cooperation. According to a Gallup poll, in early 1989, 70% of Americans showed favorable or very favorable feelings towards China.

As for the international situation, the global pattern of bi-polarity to multi-polarity is more pronounced and fixed. In 1969, President Nixon suggested the idea of the "five powers" of the international system: the U.S., the Soviet Union, Europe, China, and Japan. With China joining the U.N. as one of the five permanent member states, its international status and role cannot be overlooked.

Meanwhile, China contrived to crawl out of the diplomatic disorder during the Cultural Revolution. As the domestic situation became stable, the Chinese economy began to soar. While adhering to independence in foreign policy, China lifted the curtain of reform and opening up. It actively blended into the international community, carefully managed its relations with the U.S., introduced advanced technology and management experience, and vigorously developed productive forces. In 2001, China joined the W.T.O. and welcomed explosive economic growth. Since the reform and opening up, China has witnessed rapid development for over forty years, becoming the second-largest economy after the U.S. It is increasingly apparent that it will catch up with and surpass the U.S.

Of course, there have also been some intractable crises between the two powers in the second thirty years. But these crises were under a single issue, and both parties were willing to manage and control them. The heads of state and senior officials of the two resolved the crises in a relatively short time, thus enabling the Sino-U.S. relations to sustain challenges. But generally, in the second thirty years of Sino-U.S. relations, China made continuous efforts to join and blend into the U.S.-led economic order, thus improving its global strength and status.

The Third Thirty Years

After the 2008 financial crisis, Sino-U.S. relations entered a stage of adjustment. Having survived the shocks of the previous decade, Sino-U.S. relations walked into the third thirty years. However, in the third thirty years, especially after Trump became president, the U.S. has accelerated and strengthened its suppression of China as an adversary.

Although in the second thirty years, the U.S. briefly regarded China as an adversary and made it difficult for China on a series of matters. Comparatively, China's economy was still not strong enough, despite its rapid growth during the Bush administration (2001.01–2009.01). In 2000, the G.D.P. of China was just US$ 1.211346 trillion, while that of the U.S. reached US$ 10.287479 trillion. The former was 11.78% of the latter. In 2008, the G.D.P. of China climbed to US$ 4.600589 trillion, while that of the U.S. was US$ 14.718582 trillion. The former was 31.26% of the latter.

In 2016, before Trump took office, the G.D.P. of China had reached US$ 11.194752 billion, while that of the U.S. was US$ 18.624475 billion. The former rose to 60.11% of the latter. This development state has triggered great vigilance and concern in the U.S. At this rate of development, by around 2030, the G.D.P. of China will surpass that of the U.S. and become the world's largest. This gives the U.S. a solid incentive to suppress China.

Historically, since the end of World War II, the opening of the ultimate consumer market in the U.S. has become the source of American economic power, and the success of the East Asian model was primarily based on such an international economic division of labor. In the closed fields such as finance, currency, the military, and technology, once the U.S. believes that its competitors are catching up, it will take comprehensive measures to suppress them. In the 1980s, the economic war between Japan and the U.S. was ignited by the increase in Japan's G.D.P. and by the strong trend that Japan was catching up in specific technological fields, like semiconductors. Thus, in the late Obama administration, the domestic attitude toward China has drastically changed. After Trump took office, the U.S. has, step by step, strengthened its countermeasures.

In the 2017 National Security Strategy of the United States of America, China was positioned as its primary strategic rival. The Indo-Pacific Strategy set the course for containing and suppressing China in various fields. On August 13, 2018, Trump signed the 2019 National Defense Authorization Act, which again defined Russia and China as strategic rivals and proposed to formulate a whole-of-government strategy against China.

In recent years, although the number of Chinese students studying in the U.S. has been rising, since 2015, the increase has slowed down yearly. According to public data, in the 2017–2018 academic year, the total number of mainland Chinese students studying in the U.S. was 363,341, an increase of 3.6% compared with that of 2016–2017; in the 2018–2019 academic year, the total number was 369,548, an increase of 1.7% compared with that of 2017–2018. Academic visits have suffered more uncertainty as there were visa refusals two and three times. Personnel exchanges involve both knowledge and technology and public minds between the two countries. Cooperation and personnel exchanges between enterprises should not become national security matters nor be blocked in the name of national security. Under the vision of decoupling, the massive trade volume and frequent personnel exchanges between China and the U.S. have changed from a bond between the two to a strategic competition.

In addition, the escalating trade and technology wars have shaken economic and trade relations, which had maintained the long-term balance of Sino-U.S. relations, which have been pushed to a situation of walking on thin ice. After two years of escalating tension, in January 2020, China and the U.S. signed the *Economic and Trade Agreement Between the Government of the People's Republic of China and the Government of the United States* in Washington, U.S.A. However, the agreement did not enable Sino-U.S. relations to utter a sigh of relief. Instead, the sudden COVID-19 pandemic has pushed Sino-U.S. relations into a worse predicament.

In the face of the highly infectious COVID-19 rapidly spreading and endangering the world, the fight against the virus failed to become a buffer against the intensification of Sino-U.S. relations. Friction continues between the two sides. The virus's origin, stigma, and responding patterns have become the main disputes and outstanding differences between China and the U.S. In a way, the outbreak of COVID-19 in early 2020 added new fuel for the Trump administration to further exert pressure and decoupling. Consequently, between China and the U.S., the differences have widened and deepened at a practical level, the mutual political suspicion has intensified at the government level, and the mutual hatred has worsened at the civil level. It was salt in the wounded Sino-U.S. relations.

Cooperation over Competition

In the ongoing globalization, integration, and diversification, China and the U.S., as two major powers in the world, bear special responsibilities for world peace and development, and Sino-U.S. relations will determine the course of global politics and economy. What Sino-U.S. relations become will have a bearing on whether China can achieve the two centenary goals, on the hegemony, leadership, and global role of the U.S., on the future development of both countries, and on world peace, growth, prosperity, and progress.

Historically, after World War II, based on profound reflection on conflicts and wars, an international dispute settlement mechanism centered on the U.N. was established, and essential professional international organizations such as the International Monetary Fund (I.M.F.), the World Bank, and the W.T.O. were founded. Meanwhile, the national independence movement has been booming, the democratization of international relations, the regularization of the international order, and the transparency of international politics have become more prominent. The idea that major powers shall cooperate more instead of competing is widely recognized.

From the perspective of the international situation, although various conflicts emerge in an endless stream and many problems are difficult to address, world peace and development have always been the theme of the times. Though the trade war that Trump started has been loud, it will not bring long-term economic growth to the U.S. The confrontation and conflict between China and the U.S., like the Cold War, is not in line with the trend of the times, nor with their fundamental interests. Despite the inevitability of the competition between the two major powers, it is difficult for the competition to become a whole confrontation and conflict. Instead, cooperation in the competition must become their main move.

In addition, as China and the U.S. are the largest- and second-largest economies in the world, and permanent member states of the U.N. Security Council, they play a pivotal role in world peace, security, stability, prosperity, and progress. They should work together to address global governance problems and challenges, which is the greatest global justice. Meanwhile, suppose the world falls into chaos, where global issues keep emerging without major powers leading the governance. In that case, all countries, including China and the U.S., will suffer, and their damage may be more significant. Therefore, win-win cooperation should become the theme of the world strategy and mutual relations between China and the U.S. to maintain a long-term cooperative win-win relationship.

Although China is expected to surpass the U.S. and become the world's largest economy by the middle of this century, its comprehensive national strength is still weaker than that of the U.S. Although the G.D.P. of China in 2020 reached US$ 15.58 trillion, accounting for three-quarters of that of the U.S., the G.D.P. per capita of Chinese was only US$ 11,000, only one-sixth of that of the U.S. Compared with China, the U.S. still holds obvious advantages in higher education, technological innovation, financial management, and talent development. However, its current shortcomings are more exposed, mainly due to the problems accumulated in its system over the years. The U.S., under the raging COVID-19 pandemic, cannot fully heal its society in the short term due to its ineffective pandemic prevention and control. The current American economy relies on continuous preferential moves from the Federal Reserve. It is going through an unprecedented stage of excessive overdrafts of the U.S. dollar. As it is being over-issued, the country has become increasingly bloated, but its economy has not gained any substantial growth. And this single move of relying on the hegemony and monopoly of the U.S. dollar to export inflation to the world will not strengthen the leadership of the U.S. but further weaken it. Suppose the U.S. does not adjust its policies and focus on recovering its domestic economy and improving its comprehensive national strength as soon as possible. In that case, the hegemony of the U.S. dollar will be gone within ten years.

On the other hand, according to the law of historical development, China's present international status is similar to that of the U.S. before World War I. The most influential country in the world at that time was the U.K. The U.S. was only an emerging economic power whose political influence was not strong enough to enter the mainstream Western political system dominated by the U.K. at that time. Also, the U.S. lacked cultural confidence, and the American military was not strong enough back then. However, the

American economy was thriving and growing rapidly, propelling a great leap in military science and technology, thus laying the foundation for the U.S. to become a global leader in the future.

The raging COVID-19 pandemic has proved the difficulty for the world to be united. Just like in World War II, the world has been divided into two opposing camps, China and the U.S. When faced with an invisible opponent, the virus, we regret to see the man-made opposition in human society. The consequence of such confrontation is that the pandemic cannot be eradicated in a predictable time. However, the current globalization has entered an irreversible stage, where trade and economic exchanges make it impossible for countries to stay completely isolated. At this time, if the West, led by the U.S., fails to face and accept that China is rising objectively, it will undoubtedly negatively impact the unity and stability of human society.

Simultaneously, the widening gap between the rich and the poor, and the impact on values from Internet technology, including the intensification of racial discrimination, have deteriorated the rat race in the West to various degrees. Of course, if the U.S. can adjust its national strategy as soon as possible, namely from changing the current hegemonic strategy of expanding global domination to focusing on internal reform and governance, optimizing the various internal contradictions from social development, and continuing to absorb and attract the world's top talents and build its robust legal safeguard system, active capital atmosphere, and inclusive innovation pattern, it will stay a leader.

Political Islam generally refers to the broad political demands of Islamic religious power. It is a religious, political trend and movement. The ideology of Political Islam refers to the product of political people's political processing of Islam. By reinterpreting part of religious teachings or inventing new traditions, they package specific political propositions as religious responsibilities and guide the public's religious enthusiasm for politics. Such religious and political ideology includes "true faith," Sharia or Islamic states, and Ummah. And the ultimate goal of Political Islam is political power.

1.7 Global Governance Faces Development Challenges

The global spread of the COVID-19 pandemic has accumulated many risks, such as global economic recession, international financial market turmoil, and the broken global industrial chain. The global governance system must control it. However, the U.N. and the W.H.O., which should have played a role in global governance during the pandemic, have exposed the shortcomings of the existing global governance system in fighting the pandemic. Instead, they failed to unite various countries to effectively fight the virus.

Poor performance of the UN

From the perspective of global governance, as the world's largest, most authoritative, and universal international multilateral institution, the U.N. shoulders heavy responsibilities and plays an important role. However, the ravages of the COVID-19 pandemic around the globe have exposed the U.N.'s shortcomings and deficiencies in international cooperation and global governance, severely weakening the leadership and authority thereof.

As the most important multilateral mechanism for global governance, specialized agencies in the U.N. are committed to preventing and controlling the COVID-19 pandemic. However, the improper allocation of resources, the disconnection between theory and practice, and the disorder of global and regional linkages are the culprits for the poor performance of the U.N. in the worldwide fight against COVID-19. Thus, countries returned to the framework of nationalism. It is of great significance to the international stability in the post-COVID times, reshaping the leadership of the U.N., preventing the trend of marginalization and hollowing out, and rebuilding an effective multilateral consultation mechanism.

At the beginning of 2020, the COVID-19 pandemic broke out. In just a few months, it swept over 200 countries and regions, causing not only political, economic, and social crises but a direct blow to the global health governance system centered on the U.N. The authority, professionalism, and dominance of the U.N. have been widely questioned, and countries have returned to regionalism and nationalism to fight the pandemic.

As an international organization with the largest number of member states, the U.N. holds obvious political advantages in the fight against COVID-19. During the pandemic, it called on the international community to unite and oppose political stigma and proposed a global ceasefire and humanitarian response measures. The U.N. Security Council unanimously passed a resolution on COVID-19 in July 2020, backing up the global ceasefire initiative and humanitarian response plan proposed by the U.N. Secretary-General, and demanded that all parties in conflict with the Security Council's agenda immediately cease hostile acts, maintain a 90-day ceasefire, and ensure access to humanitarian aid and enhanced security for peacekeepers. Meanwhile, the resolution stressed the critical role of the U.N. in the global fight against the pandemic, reaffirmed a people-centered concept, and called on the international community to unite and fight the pandemic together.

At the same time, various specialized agencies of the U.N. have begun to release policy briefs continuously, offering professional and specialized guidance and advice to governments in the fight against the pandemic. For example, in June 2020, the U.N. Pandemic and the World of Work released a report stating that the COVID-19 pandemic had caused the loss of hundreds of millions of jobs around the world, and made it impossible for S.M.E.s to survive, who are essential engines of the economy, and that the young generation might become the "generation of lockdown." In November 2020, the Department of Economic and Social Affairs of the U.N. disclosed the long-term impact of the COVID-19 pandemic on poverty, arguing that the pandemic itself and the ensuing economic crisis are reversing years of achievements in alleviating poverty. Thirty-four million people have fallen into extreme poverty, which significantly undermines the global efforts to achieve the sustainable development goal of ending extreme poverty by 2020.

It is undeniable that during the pandemic, the specialized agencies of the U.N., based on systemic risk and cost-benefit analysis, have proposed to limit the flow of people in an environment with limited response capacity; taken effective measures to quarantine and treat the infected; supported the political commitment of the Chinese government, and praised its active investigation and control of the pandemic; and ensured the rapid development of diagnostic agents, antiviral drugs and other therapies for low- and middle-income countries, as well as potentially successful vaccines. They have made a positive contribution to the global response to the pandemic.

However, as the largest international organization, the shortcomings of the U.N. have been explicitly exposed in this COVID-19 pandemic. After it broke out, U.N. Secretary-General Guterres made several speeches, calling on countries to cooperate, but few responded. In specific practices, the excessive "politicization" and "securitization" of the COVID-19 pandemic have impeded the global governance of the pandemic. Specifically, due to the political struggle between major powers, the specific resolutions of the Security Council have been challenging to implement. In particular, as a leading power, the U.S. has changed from the main driver of AIDS securitization to the only roadblock to cooperation in fighting the COVID-19 pandemic. Its unilateralism and practice of buck-passing have harmed the U.N.'s international cooperation practice in response to the COVID-19 pandemic.

On the other hand, the more important reason is the problems of the U.N. itself. Its outdated governance system, serious bureaucracy and corruption, and slow reforms have severely weakened the leadership and credibility, preventing it from playing its due role in addressing global public problems.

The W.H.O.'s Inability to Fight the Pandemic

In 1946, the U.N. founded the W.H.O., based on the three major international health organizations. Next, it formulated the International Health Regulations (I.H.R.) in 1951, expanding the management scope from the initial control of infectious diseases to public health.

After the end of the Cold War, due to the challenges of globalization of diseases, especially the new infections of AIDS, SARS, HINI influenza, Ebola, COVID-19, and "super bacteria," pandemics strike more frequently. The W.H.O. continued to expand and approved the amended I.H.R. (2005) at the 58th World Health Assembly in 2005, establishing its leadership in responding to global public health crises.

In particular, having learned a lesson from SARS in 2003, for countries to prevent and control the occurrence of similar outbreaks effectively, the W.H.O. Director-General will seek the opinion of the Emergency Committee to decide whether a specific incident constitutes a public health emergency of international concern (P.H.E.I.C.), to which each member state has the legal responsibility to respond quickly.

When a regional outbreak is declared a P.H.E.I.C., the W.H.O. needs to issue an interim recommendation on the health measures that countries should take for people, goods, and transportation, coordinate global human and material resources, and provide guidance and assistance to regions where a P.H.E.I.C. occurs when necessary, such as raising external aid funds.

Since its establishment, the governance performance of the W.H.O. has made relatively satisfying achievements in response to regional small-scale outbreaks or single diseases. Since 2009, it has declared a total of six P.H.E.I.C.s. In the absence of a significant global pandemic, the W.H.O. has performed well in small local outbreaks, and the level of compliance and cooperation of various countries has been high.

However, in managing this large-scale COVID-19 pandemic, the W.H.O. was exposed to slow response, low efficiency, and weak capability. On January 30, 2020, W.H.O. Director-General Dr. Tedros Adhanom Ghebreyesus stated that as per the I.H.R., given the surge in confirmed cases in other countries, W.H.O. had reached a consensus after discussion that the outbreak met the criteria of a P.H.E.I.C., and therefore it was declared a P.H.E.I.C. However, in the fight against COVID-19, the W.H.O. has been frequently caught in the whirlpool of disputes due to its failure to coordinate the relations between major powers.

First, former U.S. President Donald J. Trump publicly accused the W.H.O. of being China-centric in the pandemic prevention and control and announced on April 14, 2020, that the U.S. would suspend the payment of membership dues to the W.H.O. Then, Chairman of the U.S. Senate Committee on Homeland Security Ronald Johnson also announced an independent investigation of the W.H.O. and its Director-General Dr. Tedros Adhanom Ghebreyesus, urging them to provide relevant information. Regardless of the purpose of these accusations, they have weakened the professionalism and credibility of the W.H.O. and hindered it from playing a part in the fight against the pandemic.

Meanwhile, different regions and countries have not been able to agree on whether to enter a state of emergency and what response measures to take. Some have imposed partial city lockdowns, some have chosen partial state lockdowns, some have gone with total state lockdowns, and some have turned to herd immunity. The W.H.O.'s inability to coordinate various regions and countries effectively has exacerbated the chaos and disorder in response to the COVID-19 pandemic and made it more difficult for the U.N. to perform global health governance.

The critical factors to the W.H.O.'s failure to effectively lead the various countries to fight against the pandemic are its own bureaucracy, corruption, and unprofessionalism. Among the recently exposed scandal of the W.H.O.'s assistance to some places, there have been staff who sexually assaulted local women and children. This is the greatest disgrace to the W.H.O., directly, leading to the collapse of its credibility.

From Challenge to Response

Global governance is the cooperative governance of state and non-state actors that is free from state-centered and socially-centered ideas. Without a unified global government, the U.N., an international intergovernmental organization exclusive to sovereign states, has naturally become a vital force in global public governance. Moreover, with the deepening of globalization into a "global village," it is even more necessary for the U.N. and other international organizations to perform better.

The U.N. and its international agencies are more responsible for coordinating global development, and their corresponding powers to deal with problems should also be strengthened. This is the law of the development of things. The COVID-19 pandemic has exposed the flaws and inadequacies of the U.N. Without a global coordination mechanism that keeps pace with the times, the U.N. and its international agencies are less efficient. And the test the U.N. faces is also a common test for the international community.

In the post-COVID times, if the U.N. wants to remain valuable and influential, it must reform the original system, improve the prevention and control system, and build a greater coping capability. Taking the institutional design features of the W.H.O. as an example, the institutional design model of W.H.O., similar to that of most international agencies, is a global cooperation model that requires all parties to abide by the anarchic institutional strategy. When W.H.O. declares an outbreak in a specific region as a P.H.E.I.C., member states should respond quickly, take sanitary measures for people, goods, and transportation, and coordinate human and material resources to raise aid funds and provide guidance and assistance to the affected region.

However, the inherent institutional design of the W.H.O. is unable to sustain the blow of the COVID-19 pandemic, especially when a large number of medical resources, medical equipment, and anti-pandemic materials are highly concentrated in developed countries. The W.H.O. can only provide limited professional guidance without being able to respond in time. As a result, in the middle and late stages of the COVID-19 pandemic, when most developed countries were overwhelmed and unable to help the developing countries, the weakness of W.H.O.'s governance capacity was further exposed. In the post-COVID times, as a representative of the international public health system and a global institutional framework accepted by member states, the U.N. must adhere to institutional cooperation while reforming its institutional design, which is the key to the W.H.O.'s response to COVID-19.

For example, by improving international law and promoting corresponding institutional building, the W.H.O. can have executable power similar to the W.T.O.'s trade dispute settlement mechanism so that it plays a more authoritative and effective role in determining the criteria for pandemic case confirmation, publishing statistics of data and information, supervising the implementation of domestic pandemic prevention and control measures in various countries, and mediating their conflicts in those measures.

Simultaneously, it is necessary to give greater financial support to the W.H.O. According to the W.H.O. budget proposal for 2018-2019, only US$ 554 million was allocated to deal with global health emergencies. However, as the U.S. still owes the W.H.O. about US$ 300 million in dues and has sharply cut its financial support to it in 2021 from US$ 123 million in 2020 to US$ 58 million, it is more difficult for the W.H.O. to maintain its normal operations. Therefore, a punishment system should be established to deter countries from refusing or delaying the payment of W.H.O. membership dues.

Secondly, in the ongoing global prevention and control of the COVID-19 pandemic, regional international organizations have played a key role in information sharing, resource allocation, organization, and coordination. Therefore, how cooperating with them closely is a crucial test of the U.N.'s ability to contain the COVID-19 pandemic. However, the truth is whether it is a pandemic judgment or specific measures, the world's only public health governance organization, the W.H.O., lacks the pertinence and flexibility of regional organizations such as the E.U. and ASEAN.

For example, in the practice of promoting the construction of a global public health governance system, ASEAN, China, Japan, and South Korea (the "10+3" mechanism) have held a special anti-pandemic meeting of leaders, a unique video conference of senior health development officials, a video conference of state health ministers, a special video conference of economic and trade ministers, and so on, to coordinate the funds, materials, and personnel of various countries. They have united to curb the spread of the pandemic, improve the level of public health governance, and promote the recovery of regional economic growth. Their practices and experiences are good examples for other regions and should be promoted worldwide.

In comparison, due to the differences in the severity of the COVID-19 pandemic in different regions and the objective needs of pandemic prevention such as working from home and city-state lockdowns, it is difficult for homogeneous international organizations represented by the U.N. to act promptly. There are sometimes delayed actions and governance failures. Therefore, in the post-COVID-19 times, the U.N. should enhance its leadership in agenda-setting and project planning coordination and reshape its global public health product supplier role. And its top priority is to set up differentiated pandemic prevention tasks through close cooperation with regional international organizations and allocate resources reasonably according to the development characteristics and direction of the COVID-19 pandemic in different regions.

Finally, the intensified strategic competition among major powers is another important cause that has prevented the U.N. and its related agencies from effectively responding to the COVID-19 pandemic. For a long time, the attitudes of major powers towards global governance and the degree of cooperation between them have been the key to the total exertion of the U.N.'s governance capacity. In recent years, the international situation has undergone dramatic changes. The financial crisis and populism have hit the old international order hard. Due to the intensified competition among major powers, especially the whole-government, all-around, global, and multi-field competition between China and the U.S., it is difficult for a new international order to take shape in the short term. Therefore, the outbreak of the COVID-19 pandemic has made the already fragile global governance system more stagnant.

The structure of international power and interests is being divided and reorganized, and the time when the international order lacks a dominant force is around the corner. The strategic competition among major powers will also affect whether the U.N. can continue to be useful. And whether China will be respected and recognized by Western democratic countries will be an essential factor in whether the U.N. can continue to be useful.

When China's economy surpasses the U.S. and tops the world, its influence will attract more and more international organizations and institutions, including some emerging organizations and influential organizations of the U.N., to relocate to China, and its role in the U.N. will have greater weight.

It is an unstoppable trend that the further improvement of China's economic strength is bound to promote its comprehensive national strength. China is the only country whose civilization has never ceased to exist, and its culture contains profound experience in international leadership. The U.S. is only over 200 years old. It undoubtedly possesses strong innovation and modern social governance capabilities but lacks experience in failure and conflict conciliation. When competing with a major power like China with 5,000 years of national governance experience, the experience of the U.S. will obviously be insufficient.

Suppose China and the U.S. cannot face each other objectively, accept each other objectively, and keep cooperation and competition. In that case, it will harm the entire human society, and the leadership of the U.N. will be weakened. It is foreseeable that in this century, the U.N. can play the role of a global leader and whether it can become the chief umpire of international multilateral negotiations as before depending on the development of Sino-U.S. relations.

Similarly, in times of globalization, a virus anywhere on the planet can spread quickly and cause far more damage than ever. As the world's largest, most authoritative, and universal global multilateral institution, the U.N. plays a crucial role in global governance. In the post-COVID times, the U.N. should contribute more to building a community with a shared future.

But unfortunately, after over 70 years of development, the U.N., founded on October 24, 1945, and the W.H.O., founded on April 7, 1948, have accumulated a growing number of problems. The COVID-19 pandemic has only accelerated the burst of the issues. There is a mountain of problems in the U.N., such as excessive bureaucracy, corruption, sexual abuse of women and children, lack of transparency in the use of funds, insufficient support for developing countries (especially for poor countries), and lack of decisive execution on some critical matters... These problems have made the U.N. less useful but become a battlefield for major powers and a stage for diplomatic performances. It is increasingly difficult for the U.N. to unite countries worldwide to address major problems and challenges to humanity jointly.

There is certain representativeness in China's proposals on the reform of the U.N. China believes that such reform should be conducive to promoting multilateralism, improving the authority and efficiency of the U.N., as well as its ability to handle new threats and challenges. The reform should uphold the purposes and principles of the U.N. Charter, especially sovereign equality, non-interference in internal affairs, peaceful settlement of disputes, and strengthening of international cooperation; it should be all-round and in many fields; it should make achievements in both security and development; in particular, it should reverse the trend of "security over development" in the work of the U.N., increase investment in development, and promote the implementation of the millennium development goals; it should meet the demands and concerns of all member states, especially the developing states, to the greatest extent possible; it should promote democracy, make full consultations, and strive to reach the broadest consensus; it should be carried out step-by-step to maintain and improve the unity of the U.N. member states; for agreed recommendations, the U.N. should make decisions as soon as possible to implement them; on major issues with remaining differences, it should be cautious, continue consultations, strive for broad consensus, and refrain from artificially setting time limits or forcibly pushing for decisions.

It is foreseeable that if the U.N. organization fails to carry out profound reforms as soon as possible, the world will not be able to cooperate better under its mediation, and it will have a weaker role and value as a global coordinator faster after 2035.

CHAPTER 2

The Digital Revolution Breeds Economic Changes

WHILE THE COVID-19 PANDEMIC INFLICTS HEAVY LOSSES ON THE GLOBAL economy, stirring up a crisis, it has also bred new opportunities, accelerating the development of the digital economy and pushing society into a new era of digitalization. Human society is marching from the physical world into the digital world. Although the popularization of computers, smartphones, and network technologies has already altered people's lives and consumption habits, the digital economy is no simple industrial revolution. It has innovated the way of value creation, redefined the process of value distribution, and resolved the obvious clash with the old ideas and the old order rooted in the traditional economy. The COVID-19 pandemic has forced people to completely separate from the physical world for the first time and reflect on the causes and effects of the real world, which may accelerate the formation of a social order and a moral culture adapted to the digital economy.

General information technology that is centered on digital technology is promoting a new round of technological revolution and industrial transformation on a global scale, which has a profound impact on value creation. The digital economy has become the primary form of international economic development and the main driving force for future economic growth. It is paramount, and there are more and more voices discussing digitization and the digital economy.

Currently, various industries and enterprises around the world are undergoing a digital transformation. By leveraging digital assets, developing new applications, expanding new capabilities, and pioneering new ideas, new areas of innovation are explored faster, more efficiently, and more reliably. From small increments comes abundance. Every small step forward in digitalization will significantly impact overall economic development. As a result, the true digital revolution is coming, and the global economy, trade relations, international structure, and even the monetary order will usher in a historical turning point.

2.1 Faster Occurrence of Cashlessness

In the raging COVID-19 pandemic, as banknotes might spread the virus, many countries have successfully set forth a banknote disinfection policy and advocated reducing the use of cash. Meanwhile, unprecedented mass social distancing has accelerated the popularization of electronic cash and e-payments. Because of these circumstances, cashlessness is happening faster.

From Paper Money to Digital Money

Before discussing the changes in payment modes led by currency changes, it is necessary to understand the history of changes in currencies. Before the emergence of currency, initial consumption was a decentralized institutional arrangement of bartering. However, human beings' economic activities and trade scope were greatly restricted due to the extremely low transaction efficiency, the difficulty in coupling supply and demand, and the lack of a unified value measurement standard. Therefore, precious metals such as gold and silver were used as currency.

Gold and silver were one of the first forms of currency. Professor Natacha Postel-Vinay, who teaches monetary and financial history at the London School of Economics, pointed out that currency is a relatively new invention that represents the fundamental changes in human society.

The first recorded use of currency was in ancient Iraq and Syria during the Babylonian civilization around 3000 BCE. In Babylonian times, people used large chunks of silver, which were measured according to a standard weight called the shekel. From Babylon came the first records of prices, by priests at the Temple of Merodach, as well as the first books of accounts and the first debts.

When Babylon gathered many of the basic elements needed for a monetary economy, including regular testing of the purity of silver and the trust in a king or government to guarantee the value of the currency, a currency with the backing of national credit that was a pure fiduciary currency was born.

Paper money was the first leap of credit money from specific objects to abstract symbols. China's earliest use of paper money was in the Tang Dynasty (618–907 CE). Paper money at the time was a privately issued note of credit or exchange, but it wasn't until the 17th century that Europe began to embrace this idea.

The development of technology has blessed the evolution of currency. As a result, people have entered an era of more convenient payment. The credit card was invented in 1946 by John Biggins of the Flatbush National Bank in Brooklyn, New York. Subsequently, it was promoted in the U.S. to traveling salesmen to use during business trips. On June 29, 1966, the British Barclays Bank issued the U.K.'s first credit card.

In October 1979, the Guangzhou Branch of the Bank of China took the lead in issuing the Visa credit card on behalf of the Bank of East Asia in Hong Kong. That was when the credit card entered the Chinese market. After that, the bank card business has developed to a certain extent. All major banks have issued their bank cards. To improve cardholders' usage scenarios and experience, they are equipped with corresponding acceptance equipment, the Point of Sale (P.O.S.) machine. Therefore, card-swiping became high-end consumer behavior in China in the 1980s and 1990s.

Soon, the limitations of P.O.S. machines became apparent. They crowded counters and operated on different rates, which led to a surge in business owner's costs, difficulty in accounting management, and limited acceptance of cardholders, thus violating their rights and interests. Therefore, in June 1993, the State Council of China launched various card-based application system projects to develop electronic money and a focus on the application of electronic money. From that point, the era of UnionPay began.

When UnionPay and major banks were developing rapidly in the offline market, online payment took another road with the rapid development of the mobile Internet: payment institutions. In 2003, on the banks of the West Lake in Hangzhou, Alipay, as a division of Taobao, launched an online secured transaction service for Taobao, which changed the pattern of the Chinese payment market and profoundly affected the development of the payment market in the next decade.

Currency is another important invention of human beings in addition to language. After bartering, and the gold and silver standard, credit currency was a giant leap in the history of currency. While paper money was the first leap of credit currency from specific items to abstract symbols, a digital currency based on blockchains, artificial intelligence, cloud computing, and big data is the second leap of credit currency from paper form to paperlessness.

Unchangeable Future Trends

Undoubtedly, from a historical point of view, we have reason to believe that as everything has a cycle of birth, development, and death, it is entirely possible for paper money to disappear soon. The change from paper money to digital currency is bound to happen. In fact, as early as May 2014, Israel announced the abolition of cash transactions, and most transactions in many countries are now paid through electronic devices.

Compared with digital currency, paper money has many drawbacks and great security risks: first, it is a huge waste of resources. The service life of banknotes is the shortest compared to other forms of money. A banknote is no longer used after three years of circulation. Generally, the lifespan of a banknote is 18–20 months. When it is not used for a long time, buried in the ground, or left alone for a long time, it will mold and rot, which is why countries have to keep issuing new banknotes.

Second, because paper money has been used and circulated in people's hands for a long time, it has become the most likely medium to spread bacteria and viruses. The abundant bacteria on the banknotes are dangerous to human health and life. As we have learned from COVID-19, though it is not proven that the use of cash can spread the virus, the strong liquidity of paper money indeed makes it easy to carry various bacterial pathogens. Instead, non-cash payment reduces the risk of human contact and the spread of bacteria during the circulation of banknotes and impedes disease transmission to a certain extent.

Third, it is not easy to carry large-denomination banknotes. Instead, they are a great safety hazard. The tangibility of paper money and the fact that it must be carried around make it the easiest target for all kinds of criminals. However, ordinary criminals cannot easily steal electronic money with high-tech security without the help of high-tech means and special methods. The security of digital currency is much higher than that of paper money.

In contrast to the unavoidable drawbacks and great security risks of paper money, digital currency has exhibited its unique advantages: for the government, digital currency is a powerful tool for anti-corruption; for enterprises, financial fraud becomes impossible for society, it leaves financial crimes nowhere to hide. Digital currency has a relatively secure cryptographic system. Especially with the emergence of chip bank cards, the security performance of digital currency will continue to improve. And electronic money has a much longer lifespan and greater durability than cash.

In addition, the central bank's digital currency, endorsed by the sovereignty, embedded with programmable design, and unique with precise drip irrigation from top to bottom, is coupled with the blockchain due to its traceable characteristics throughout its entire lifespan. It will reconstruct the exchange system and stimulate the new potential of the digital economy. And the digital currency is focused on fitting the basic properties of currency and making up for the disconnection between the old currency system and the new digital economy.

Under the conditions of a developed commodity economy, currency has five functions: to measure value, means of circulation means of storage, means of payment, and world currency. In the future operating system of the digital economy era, the new generation of international currency still needs to perform the above functions. Therefore, only by strengthening the integration with the digital economy's development model can the digital economy's growth potential be brought into play. Since digital currency adopts electronic payment, it is convenient to be widely used in the world in digital form, thus meeting the requirement to be a world currency itself.

In 2018, the international authorities Committee on Payments and Market Infrastructures (C.P.M.I.) and Market Committee (M.C.) defined central bank digital currency as a new variant of central bank currency different from physical cash or central bank reserves or settlement accounts. Based on the four dimensions of the issuer (central bank or non-central bank), form (digital currency or traditional paper money), accessibility (open or restricted), and technology, the digital currency of global central banks is divided into general-purpose digital currency and wholesale digital currency.

The central banks of various countries have reached a consensus on the importance of digital currency to the digital economy era. Many central banks are studying blockchain and encrypted digital currencies and conducting technical tests. Some have officially set forth relevant digital currency issuance and payment policies, such as the European Central Bank (E.C.B.), Riksbank, Bank of Canada, Bank of Japan, and the Monetary Authority of Singapore. The Central bank of Uruguay has piloted a central bank digital currency (C.B.D.C.) on a limited scale; The central bank of the Philippines supports a private sector digital fiat currency (D.F.C.) for payment under a regulatory sandbox system.

Central bank digital currency is bound to happen in the digital economy era because it can provide the public with a safer and more liquid payment method. As it is endorsed by national credit, it can greatly reduce the operating cost of fiat currency, improve payment efficiency, and facilitate cross-border payments.

From the perspective of application scenarios, human beings' earliest means of exchange was barter; later, shells were used as currency. However, current research shows that over half of consumers prefer digital payments. In a survey of 17 European countries in 2019, the E.C.B. found that the vast majority of consumers tended to continue to use digital payment or further increase their use of it after the COVID-19 pandemic is over.

According to McKinsey & Co's July 2020 report, the early currencies were copper, gold, and silver. Before the advent of paper money, exchanges between people were still exchanges of physical objects. In the digital currency era, currency becomes a string of encrypted characters, which are carried by the applications on a mobile phone. The exchange can be completed during a trade simply by scanning the QR code or via near-field communication. It is worth mentioning that, according to the information disclosed by People's Bank of China, its D.C.E.P. (digital currency electronic payment) adopts the dual offline payment method. The payment can be completed when both parties are offline and without an Internet connection. This reflects the advantages of cash payment and makes up for the inconvenience of WeChat and Alipay that there must be an Internet connection for the payment to be completed.

Andrew Bailey, Governor of the Bank of England, also stated recently that the demand for non-cash payments in the U.K. is rising significantly. Affected by the COVID-19 pandemic and social distancing, the volume of cash withdrawals in the U.K., which had already been shrinking, continued to shrink. It fell by 60% in April 2020 compared to the same period the year before. Even in July, when social distancing was lifted, cash withdrawals remained low, down 40% from a year earlier. Victoria Cleland, Executive Director for Banking, Payments, and Innovation at the Bank of England, stated recently that the scale of global cross-border payments is expected to rise to US$ 250 trillion in 2027, a bump of $100 trillion from 10 years ago. However, such large-scale cross-border payments face hindrances such as cost, speed, availability, and transparency.

Finally, digital currency also provides a meaningful way to balance technological innovation and contemporary governance issues. While the technological revolution has brought about a massive leap in economic and social efficiency, it may have a major impact on contemporary governance models. The use of unofficial digital currency represented by Bitcoin in drugs, guns, ammunition, money laundering, and so on warns us to keep an eye on technological innovation's negative impact and risks.

In general, compared with cash, even if digital currency still faces the negative impact of technological innovation, cashlessness is inevitable. It is foreseeable that by around 2035, the cashless model will be mainstream in all advanced economies.

2.2 The Impact of Digital Currency Diversification

With the increasing popularity of mobile payments worldwide, more and more central banks have begun actively researching and experimenting with issuing digital currency. According to the Bank for International Settlements statistics, at least 17 countries' central banks are actively exploring digital currency issuance, and some have even implemented or are implementing related digital currency issuance trial programs.

Among them, China is also at the forefront of the research and exploration of the central bank's issuance of digital currency with the help of its advantages in the mobile payment industry and financial technology. As early as April 2020, the People's Bank of China disclosed that it was ready to issue D.C.E.P. and had already started trials in many locations.

Indeed, while the application of digital currency by central banks around the world is accelerating, it will inevitably face the challenge of the impact of digital currency diversification. How to meet the challenges is a road that digital currency has never taken.

Money Denationalization Comes True

In his book *Denationalization of Money*, Austrian economist Friedrich August von Hayek proposed the idea that the government's monopoly of the money supply should be broken. Instead, private institutions should supply different currencies. The birth of Facebook's encrypted digital currency Libra in 2019 marked the beginning of a new era of digital currency, as well as that von Hayek's vision of money denationalization and diversified currency has gradually come true.

Shortly after the birth of Libra, I.M.F. President Christine Lagarde also stated that the I.M.F. planned to launch a global digital currency—I.M.F. Coin based on the S.D.R. mechanism. So, digital currency has been officially recognized and supported by international authoritative financial institutions, and more and more official institutions have begun to re-examine the development trend of blockchain and digital currency.

In February 2019, JPMorgan Chase released its own digital currency, the J.P.M. coin, for inter-institutional clearing. Meanwhile, I.B.M. announced its own cross-border payment blockchain system, World Wire. On July 25, 2020, a U.S. federal court officially recognized virtual currencies such as Bitcoin as a lawful currency of the country. This also means that the integration of technology and finance and the trend of digital currency and virtual assets have become unstoppable.

Though Markus Rodlaue stressed that Libra would work with the Federal Reserve and other central banks to ensure that it does not interfere with the central bank's monetary policy and is subject to the supervision of legal institutions, the endless emergence of encrypted digital currencies, whether legal or private, will inevitably affect the global central bank's money supply and money creation, the effectiveness of monetary policy and financial supervision to varying degrees.

Undoubtedly, the digital currency represented by Libra is already ahead of the central banks. In the digital currency era, the statistical caliber and scope of the global central bank money supply need to be adjusted. The central bank's total money supply is no longer the unit of accounting in economic activities but a combination of encrypted assets and units of account. Moreover, monetary policy instruments are not limited to interest rates and deposit reserve ratios, and a series of new monetary policy indicators such as cryptocurrency interest rates will appear.

Digital cryptocurrencies may partially weaken the central bank's leading role in monetary policy because they will inevitably have a certain crowding-out effect on the circulation of traditional currencies. The quantity and speed of currency circulation will affect the currency multiplier. The crowding-out effect depends on the competition among legal digital currency, private digital currency, and traditional currency. The result of this competition is manifested in the exchange ratio between legal tender and private money.

Obviously, with the rise of various Internet businesses and the popularization of blockchain, blockchain-based digital currency has replaced the current legal tender's credit function to a large extent. In the future, some commercial entities will issue various digital currencies based on their ecosystems, and the alliance model between different commercial entities will allow the digital currencies among them to be effectively circulated. And the consequence will be that the number of digital currency types will exceed that of national currencies.

Indeed, the operation system of the central bank-commercial bank dual currency model fully considers the dredging of monetary policy interest rate transmission channels. The People's Bank of China's D.C.E.P. only replaces traditional legal tender such as banknotes and coins, which is conducive to improving the controllability and testability of money supply. It is foreseeable that with the popularization of digital currency technology and the further popularization of Internet lifestyles such as the metaverse, the competition between money denationalization and legal tender will become an important issue that challenges governments in the upcoming ten years. In addition to the competition between the digital currency making of the Internet platform and the legal tender so far, there will also be a diversified currency competition between non-nationalized currencies (private currencies), digital currencies, and traditional currencies in the future.

Digital Currency Intensifies Competition Between Legal Tenders

The central bank's digital currency is focused on fitting the basic properties of the currency and making up for the disconnection between the old monetary system and the new digital economy. However, suppose the advanced nature of the central bank digital currency is limited to expanding the payment system's boundary, extending the pricing means, or evolving functions. In that case, its impact and significance will obviously stir up an increasingly heated discussion on a global scale. Therefore, the impact of currency diversification cast by the birth of a number of central bank digital currencies and commercial currencies not only ignites the competition between money denationalization and legal tender but intensifies the competition between legal tenders.

As E.C.B. President Christine Lagarde put it, currency is a symbol of sovereignty while it facilitates transactions. Moreover, the issuance of central bank digital currency is of great significance to developed economies in terms of payment security, financial stability, and the supervision of non-sovereign digital currencies. For emerging market economies, it matters greatly in terms of payment efficiency and financial inclusion and has an incomparable advantage over the traditional method in dealing with the crisis of exchange rate depreciation. This is also why major economies have activated the central bank digital currency program and participated in the currency competition.

For example, there is "one currency, two databases, and three centers" of the People's Bank of China. Among them, one currency refers to D.C.E.P. only, a legal digital currency endorsed by the credit of the People's Bank of China. It is equal to the RMB; the two databases are the issuance database and the commercial bank database, which make up a two-tier operation system of D.C.E.P., that is, People's Bank of China manages the issuance database, accepts D.C.E.P. with commercial banks, and does not directly face the public.

The three centers include the certification center, the registration center, and the big data analysis center. The registration center records the bank statement and ownership, while the certification center confirms the identity. The two independently ensure the anonymity of D.C.E.P. transactions. For suspicious transaction records, only the People's Bank of China has the ultimate authority to track them, which can effectively curb money laundering and other illegal transactions. The above-mentioned controllable anonymity continues the characteristics of paper currency transactions while preventing digital currency from participating in illegal acts. It plays a vital role in enhancing market competitiveness and maintaining market discipline.

European countries represented by Norway, Sweden, and others issue digital currencies to use as a supplement to legal tender to maintain the stability of the operating monetary system. In addition, there are some petrodollar countries. For example, to break the U.S. dollar blockade and depend less on it, Venezuela issues a digital currency that can be converted into legal tender or gold as a reserve instrument to stabilize currency value and the normal operation of the domestic economy.

As the pioneer of the central bank digital currency and electronic payment system, China's related R&D pilot programs, and their external effects have attracted wide attention from all parties. Preparing the People's Bank of China for digital currency dates back to 2014. With the support of Zhou Xiaochuan, Governor of the People's

Bank of China, it assembled a special research group to issue legal digital currency. And the news of digital currency development has continued to be disclosed over the years. In November 2019, Fan Yifei, Deputy Governor of the People's Bank of China, stated that digital currency has basically completed top-level design, standard formulation, functional R&D, and joint debugging and testing. It is expected that it will start to use digital currency in 2022. Compared with other countries, based on the rich practical experience of electronic payment, the People's Bank of China's digital currency R&D is fast. In the global competition for central bank digital currency, China is at the forefront.

On August 14, 2020, the Ministry of Commerce of the People's Republic of China issued the *Overall Plan for Comprehensively Deepening the Pilot Program of Innovative Development of Service Trade*. Regarding comprehensively deepening the pilot program, specific measures, and division of responsibilities for the innovative development of service trade, it proposed that Beijing-Tianjin-Hebei, the Yangtze River Delta, Guangdong-Hong Kong-Macao Greater Bay Area, and eligible regions in the central and western China carry out the digital RMB pilot program. The People's Bank of China formulates policy safeguard measures; Shenzhen, Chengdu, Suzhou, Xiong'an New Area, and other places perform the pilot program first. It will be expanded to other regions if the pilot turns out well. On September 14th, Fan Yifei, Deputy Governor of the People's Bank of China, published an article online on baidu.com called *Some Considerations About the Central Bank Digital Currency*, which the outside world saw as the most official "spoiler" about D.C.E.P.

Under the catalyst of the COVID-19 pandemic, the infrastructure construction of D.C.E.P. has been further accelerated. D.C.E.P. will likely take place earlier than expected. Around this revolutionary instrument, the People's Bank of China is expected to take the lead in completing the upgrade and transformation of the traditional monetary policy system.

On the one hand, based on built-in functions such as targeted use and smart contracts, D.C.E.P. is expected to become a powerful structural policy instrument to achieve accurate currency delivery and promote capital flow to the short-board areas on the supply side. On the other hand, based on the tracking function, D.C.E.P. is expected to provide the People's Bank of China with more detailed capital flow and economic cycle information, thereby optimizing the timing and strength of aggregate policy instruments and reducing policy transmission losses by lowering financial supervision costs. This means that China's monetary policy will stay relatively calm and active in the face of interest rate cuts by global central banks. The Sino-U.S. interest margin gap is expected to remain comfortable for a long time and support the RMB exchange rate.

In addition, as China's new economy enterprises go overseas and their corresponding digital payment system extends globally, D.C.E.P. is expected to give full play to its first-mover advantage as a central bank digital currency and occupy a leading position in the payment, settlement, and pricing functions of the global new economy. As a result, the relationship chain of RMB-DCEP-global new economic resources is expected to be opened up and continue to be consolidated. The RMB will become one of the key instruments for efficient transactions and resource allocation in the new global economy.

In fact, with the outbreak of World War I as a predisposing cause, human society had officially transitioned from the gold standard to the credit currency system, which has been over a hundred years. After the end of World War II, the Bretton Woods System laid the foundation for the U.S. dollar to be an international currency. Even after it collapsed, the global credit currency system centered on the U.S. dollar has continued to this day, and behind it is the U.S.'s unparalleled economic and military strength for the time being.

However, such an international credit currency system centered on the U.S. dollar naturally suffers from the Triffin Dilemma: on the one hand, the U.S. relies on a trade deficit to export U.S. dollars to other countries; on the other hand, a long-term trade deficit weakens the solvency of the U.S. dollar, thus weakening its status as an international reserve currency.

Currently, the currency status of the U.S. dollar is increasingly out of balance with its real economic strength. During the COVID-19 pandemic, the Federal Reserve initiated two unconventional interest rate cuts to zero and launched open-ended, unlimited quantitative easing (Q.E.) to fill the black hole of U.S. dollar liquidity. Though the short-term solution solves the urgent needs of the financial market, in the long term, it is imprudent. According to the World Bank and I.M.F., though the proportion of the U.S. dollar in global foreign exchange reserves still floats high at 62%, the U.S. in the global economy has dropped from 40% in 1960 to 24%.

Therefore, most countries holding U.S. dollar foreign exchange reserves may show concern about the Federal Reserve's unexpected monetary easing and instead look for a new currency replacement system. In this context, the upcoming digital currency may stand on the stage of history for the first time, innovating the way credit creation and reconstructing the international monetary order. This will also challenge the hegemony of the U.S. dollar. Therefore, it is predicted that by the middle of the 21st century, there will be at least three digital settlement and payment systems that are strong and independent worldwide.

2.3 Big Data Exchanges Replace Financial Exchanges

The COVID-19 pandemic has sped up the application of big data, promoted unprecedented innovation in science and technology worldwide, and driven historical changes in business modes and management concepts. Data resources have increasingly become an important production factor and strategic asset in human society. The ability to collect, analyze, and apply data has quickly become the center of international competition.

For the present international financial market, the financial exchanges in New York, London, and Hong Kong, known as the three major international financial centers, possess financial assets and values unmatched by other countries and regions. For other countries, having a global asset trading center is its biggest opportunity to change the positioning of themselves and their cities.

At present, when human beings and all things enter the era of big data through the Internet and the intelligence of all things, data will become a more valuable financial asset than oil and data transactions will be the next enormous international financial asset. In the face of the emerging big data exchange industry, all countries and regions are still on the same starting line. Whoever takes the lead in establishing a big data trading platform will first occupy the world's next financial trading platform›s commanding heights.

Obviously, the value of data resources is inseparable from the openness and circulation of data, that is, the establishment of data exchanges. In this background, third-party data trading platforms have emerged to meet the needs of the data market.

In China, as early as 2014, the first Chinese big data exchange platform, Beijing Zhongguancun Shuhai Big Data Exchange Platform was established in Zhongguancun (China's "Silicon Valley in northwest Beijing). After that, dozens of trading platforms were built, such as GBDEx (where Apple China's iCloud Data Center is located), Shanghai Data Exchange Corp, Chongqing Big Data Exchange, and Beibu Gulf Big Data Exchange, and developed nationwide.

Since 2020, *The Beijing Action Outline for Promoting the Innovation and Development of the Digital Economy (2020–2022)*, *Beijing Implementation Plan for Building a Digital Exchange Pilot Zone*, and the *Beijing International Big Data Exchange Establishment Implementation Pla* have been released one after another. They are a sign that China is accelerating the construction of a big data exchange infrastructure and a further step in integrating big data exchanges into the market.

The Necessity of Big Data Exchanges

The necessity of big data exchanges starts with the problems during big data transactions. Following cloud computing and the Internet of Things (IoT), that is, after people and all things are intelligentized and digitized, the vast application potential of big data and an optimistic market prospect have bred new business models and driven the formation of the big data value industry chain.

The value of big data is gradually being recognized by society, decision-making based on data science has become the common practice of governments and enterprises, and the urgency of the need for open data sharing is increasing daily. However, the commercialization of data ensues. The financialization of data assets such as data pricing and transactions has now become a predicament that hinders the commercialization of big data and financial capitalization.

On the one hand, from telecommunications, finance, and medical care to traditional manufacturing and education, and then to e-commerce and social platforms, there are abundant and extensive hidden big data resources in various countries. However, despite breakthroughs in the storage and mining of big data, there are still plenty of isolated data islands, mainly because all parties, who prioritize their own best interests, have not gathered the abundant big data. Especially in democratic countries, there is a relatively deeper awareness and larger legal conflict between personal privacy and the commercialization of big data. As a result, the big data owned by different entities are scattered in different places as fragments; thus, the dilemma of isolated data islands impedes the commercialization of big data to a certain extent.

In fact, data circulation is nothing new. Still, due to the lack of relevant laws and regulations in the big data exchange market, no matter in common law countries or civil law countries, there are no laws and regulations related to big data transactions. And it is precisely the lack of big data transaction rules, uncertain pricing standards, and asymmetric information between the two parties that lead to high transaction costs and unguaranteed data quality, which greatly hinders the flow of data assets.

Furthermore, Internet giants, governments, and large enterprises will have a stronger control over data sources, and data oligarchs will monopolize massive amounts of data. This sets barriers to free-market competition and makes it increasingly difficult to protect consumers.

On the other hand, there is a natural Arrow paradox in information economics, which was proposed in *Uncertainty and the Welfare Economics of Medical Care* by Kenneth Arrow, a Nobel-winning economist: information (data), different from general commodities, has an elusive nature. The buyer cannot determine the value of the information because he does not know the information (data) before purchase, and once the buyer knows it, he can copy it and will not buy it.

This is because the value of data is not absolutely certain. Data exhibits different market values compared with application subjects and processing and analysis techniques. From the perspective of market demand, in the data application process, the market value of the same data might vary greatly between enterprises with demand and those without. From the perspective of data processing and analysis techniques, the depth and scope of data mining and integration are different, the application range of data products formed by data varies greatly, and their market value will also show significant relative characteristics according to the application range.

Therefore, during data transaction, the data demander may overpay for the data because it is difficult to judge the data's quality and value without obtaining the data that can achieve the expected goal; the data provider also under-charges for the data due to the lack of information about the demander, not to mention their concerns about data security and data misuse.

Therefore, corresponding to the needs of the data market, there is a lack of transparent and controllable transaction bridges between a large number of data suppliers and data demanders. And there is often information asymmetry and poor communication. Therefore, where there are big data transactions with an unreasonable allocation of social resources, a big data exchange can guide the rational allocation of data resources and standardize the transaction process. Naturally, a big data exchange that promotes the flow of data to form a virtuous circle that creates new value has become a key direction that countries are paying great heed to. For various countries, this is a historical opportunity to redistribute global financial markets.

The Un-walked Road of Data Exchange

Take China as an example. China is one of the countries that started to explore big data exchanges relatively early. And 2015 was the fastest-growing year for Chinese big data exchanges. In April 2015, GBDEx opened with the support of Guiyang State-owned Assets Supervision and Administration Commission and completed its first transaction; in August, the first data exchange in central China, Wuhan Changjiang Big Data Trading, settled in Wuhan. After that, Central China Big Data Exchange, Wuhan East Lake Big Data Exchange, and Beijing-Tianjin-Hebei Data Exchange were founded one after another.

During this period, the number of big data exchanges proliferated. Their market share continued to increase, and the business scope continued to try to expand. It is worth noting that the exploration and attempts of Chinese big data exchanges have enjoyed strong support from the government, whether policy or funding.

As a third-party intermediary platform, big data exchanges have promoted the transformation from a one-to-one bilateral data market to a one-to-many or a many-to-many network data market. They have also enabled the potential commercial value of big data to be further released, gradually formed trading rules, and generated quantitative trading indexes, thus doubling the scale and efficiency of the data market. However, theory is one story, while reality is another.

Due to the promising market future of the big data industry and the relatively low barrier to entry in the early stage, many enterprises and institutions with the nature of big data exchange have been founded. Though most big data exchanges set up gratifying data trading goals at the beginning of their establishment, they have met with difficulties in actual operation. Amid the promising economic development, the data trading market has not reached the expected vitality. By investigating major data exchanges in China, it was found that after five years of operation, many big data exchanges have made few transactions and are still stuck in the stage of small-scale exploration. This situation is clearly connected to legal issues of ambiguous data ownership and risk-sharing.

Primarily, the degree and vigor of data openness and sharing by transaction entities such as the government, enterprises, and scientific research institutions affect the business scope and transaction quality of the data exchanges. In the face of huge market demand, data's commercial and social value has not been reasonably explored and utilized. The main bodies of China's data openness and sharing are concentrated in the government with big data, Internet operators, and scientific research institutions. The factors that hinder openness and sharing manifest in multiple dimensions, such as the concept of openness and sharing, a sound platform and technical support, a systematic management and supervision mechanism, and the final feedback effect of openness and sharing.

For instance, the Chinese government has been trying to establish a smart city management model based on big data. However, in actual applications, government staff at all levels still fail to understand data-based decision-making, modern governance, etc. deeply—the awareness of sharing waits to be formed. Even if most government departments have witnessed the efficiency brought by big data, they lack a mature management mechanism and, more importantly, avoid taking responsibility for mistakes in exploring a shared mechanism. On the other hand, the departments that are at the forefront of openness and sharing are confronted with technical predicaments, including problems like insufficient data maintenance and management. The barriers to openness and sharing are reflected in the fact that enterprises, for the sake of commercial interests, open little to one another during their competitions.

Therefore, to effectively motivate the participation and availability of subjects, it is first necessary to integrate structured and unstructured data to eliminate isolated data islands. Meanwhile, it is also essential to connect the internal and external data of the enterprises to eliminate data fragmentation. In addition, the participation of government, enterprises, and other entities should be enhanced with the supporting information security measures to promote data standardization and perfect transaction norms jointly. And by responding to the application needs of participants for data, the greater potential of the data trading market will be released.

Second, it isn't easy to fully release the great value of the scattered data. Specifically, in terms of data quality and validity, the ultimate manifestation of data value involves multiple links. The lack of quality and validity of original data affects the quality and accuracy of data transactions.

There are three reasons: first, most regional trading platforms are self-contained in a market without rules. Common problems such as inconsistent open formats, data dimensions, and semantics impede the smooth communication of the trading market. The second is the authenticity, integrity, consistency, and quality of the data directly determine the value of data assets.

Third, technical support still needs to be improved. Whether the data can be comprehensively collected and retrieved, whether obtained data are convenient for subsequent interaction and circulation in terms of format specifications, and whether valuable real-time data can be obtained, updated, and maintained on time will have an impact on the quality of data transactions. As data mining, analysis, and utilization deepen, it is necessary to make the data flow through reliable data transactions to revitalize the value of data. Great value can be created when it is ensured that the data continue to be analyzed and applied.

Finally, transaction security is part of safeguarding the overall security of big data. If the security of data transactions cannot be guaranteed, there will be immeasurable losses. Judging from the steps of a data transaction, first, problems in any link before the data transaction will cause the transaction to fail in the later stage, and both the data seller and the data supplier will have to bear the cost of a breach of contract. The second is the safety of the trading venue. The volume of data transactions is usually large. Without a safe trading venue, there will be illegal data transactions in the black data market. However, there is still no clear and specific management scheme for regulating the trading floor and what rules should be followed when setting the trading floor. Third, the qualifications and capabilities of data transaction subjects should also be included in the scope of security considerations.

This also means that every link before the completion of data transactions should be strictly controlled; otherwise, the scope of the impact will not be limited to individuals but spread to the society and the country, thereby threatening national security. In this regard, the big data exchange established in Beijing will face many challenges. And it is a problem that requires thorough consideration to build a big data trading system centered on a big data exchange so as to meet the needs of the development of the data market.

Judging from the current actual situation, there are mainly five difficulties:

The first is the boundary of data commercialization, that is, the boundary between data security and openness, privacy, and commercialization. There should be a boundary standard to which data is within the scope of national security, which is are within the scope of open social business, which data can be used for commercialization, and which cannot;

The second is the standard definition of data: which data should be classified and how. It is necessary to set up explicit data classification standards on how to define the boundaries and classification of data;

The third is the pricing of data, which is the problem after the definition and classification of data, that is, how to price the commercial value of such classified data;

The fourth is the data transaction mechanism and income distribution. The current data can be divided into five major categories: government data, industrial data, financial data, public service data, and personal business application data. The data transaction mechanism and income distribution of the first four are relatively simple; that is, the data owner enjoys the rights and interests of data commercialization. But the data generated by the commercial application of individuals is a major focus in the data transaction, which means that the user's personal use essentially generates this type of data, and it is the user's personal private behavior data. And it is debatable whether the commercial transaction of this type of data should allocate a part of the rights and interests to the users;

The fifth is big data legislation. Whether from the perspective of personal data privacy or commercialization, special legislation is required to define and protect boundaries and powers so that users and businesses can have clear legal rules for commercialization, and the commercial abuse of data is prevented from inflicting unwanted harm and disruption to everyday life.

From the perspective of social development, big data exchange is inevitable. Still, to truly promote the development of big data exchange, it is necessary to fundamentally solve the top-level design and system construction of the above five difficulties as soon as possible so that the healthy and orderly development of big data exchanges can be strongly ensured.

For all countries and regions, the financial data exchange that comes with the commercialization of big data is a rare historical opportunity. Whoever takes the lead from the legal and standard level will be the first to establish an international data exchange and gain a certain degree of right to speak in data trading. It is foreseeable that after the three global financial exchange centers in New York, London, and Hong Kong, by 2035, there will be three active big data exchanges in the world that are accompanied by a variety of debates on privacy ethics.

2.4 Digitization Widens Trade Borders

Digitization is changing every aspect of the world. With the rapid development of digital technologies such as the Internet, big data, cloud computing, blockchain, IoT, and artificial intelligence, the digital industries in various countries have witnessed rapid growth. In the meantime, the integration of digital technology and traditional sectors has picked up the pace, and the digital industry has begun to empower and transform traditional industries on a large scale. And digital technology and digitization are reconstructing the traditional industrial chain, value chain, and supply chain.

In this process, from barter to cash transactions and e-commerce, the form of trade has been transformed with the rapid advancement of digital technology. The COVID-19 pandemic in 2020 has sped up the development of various forms of digital trade. Software and information services, online education, online office, online medical consultation, online games, social media, and e-commerce have grown against the declining trend. The digital transformation of trade has become inevitable.

Digital Trade Empowers Traditional Trade

At present, countries and different institutions worldwide have different understandings of digital trade, which has no authoritative and precise definition on a global scale. And, as the impact of digital technology on economic trade expands, the borders touched by digital trade continue to widen.

From the perspective of commonality, digital trade can be roughly interpreted as relying on information networks and digital technology, and it is generated in cross-border R&D, production, trading, and consumption activities; with digital platforms as an important carrier, it is a new trade form that widely penetrates into various industries, fields, and links of international economics and trade; it is the sum of digital goods trade, digital service trade and cross-border data element trade with digital ordering and digital delivery as the main implementation models.

Intuitively, digital trade differs greatly from traditional trade. In the digital economy era, the entire trade process has undergone tremendous changes, unlike the traditional situation, exhibiting many new features.

First, online and electronic order capture has gradually become mainstream. In traditional trade, to reach a contract of purchase between parties involved in the trade, it often takes a long time to negotiate offline, and the transaction cost is usually high. In the era of digital trade, e-commerce has replaced traditional business forms, making it far easier for business owners to obtain orders. Tasks that used to require complex offline interactions can now be completed with just a few simple online operations, thus greatly reducing transaction costs.

Second, platforms have begun to play an increasingly important role in the trade. A traditional trade mostly unfolds independently between parties. In the era of digital trade, Internet platforms have become a vital role in the trade, and this change in the form of interaction has dramatically improved the efficiency of the entire trade process. If the trade is carried out one-to-one, many contracts related to the trade need to be drawn up separately, which will result in a sizeable contracting cost. Meanwhile, the breach of contract between enterprises is usually challenging to restrain, so the resulting disputes will greatly vex the trade participants. In addition, much trade-related supporting work also requires the input of both trade parties, which will also lead to massive economic waste. These problems are easily solved if the trade is carried out through platforms.

Trade parties can not only identify and perform contracts by following the standard process provided by the platform, thus saving unnecessary expenses, but also enjoy the risk guarantee and other supporting services provided by the platform. This makes the whole trade more convenient and more secure. More importantly, a platform makes it easier for trade participants to find partners.

Third, digitization has also significantly impacted how goods are delivered. In the era of digital trade, on the one hand, the digital content of commodities for trade will be greater, and so will the impact of digital factors on trade. Mass delivery of goods can be achieved directly by digital means. For example, the delivery of an online game is only a few hundred megabytes of data transmitted online. On the other hand, data is starting to rise as a special commodity. In the era of the digital economy, data, as an element, naturally flows in the market, including transnational markets, making it an essential product in international trade.

For example, coffee is the pillar industry of Rwanda. In the past, for Africa to complete the coffee trade, domestic companies in Rwanda had to collect coffee beans from farmers first and then look for customers from the European and American markets to make a deal. After the contract was signed, the coffee would be transported to the European and

American markets by air or sea and then repackaged, retailed, and delivered to consumers. The initiation of trade was mainly offline, the main participants of trade were enterprises, and the delivery mode was centralized. During the COVID-19 pandemic in 2020, farmers in Rwanda promoted their products using China's live streaming e-commerce. In a live streaming of Wei Ya, a Chinese influencer, it took only one second to sell out 3,000 kilograms of Gorilla's coffee beans from Rwanda.

The trade was initiated online, and Chinese consumers traded directly through the platform with coffee companies far away in Rwanda. After the contract was entered, the coffee was transported to various parts of China through logistics. All of this is in stark contrast to traditional trade.

Digital Trade Enters a New Phase

Today, people are familiar with digital trade because of the COVID-19 pandemic, but it took a long time for it to be promoted.

Twenty years ago, the world entered an era led by information technology, where traditional trade was also transformed into digital trade. So far, digital trade has undergone three stages, from trade information display platform to online trading platform, and to trade industry chain comprehensive service platform, and is moving towards the stage of a business operating system of digital trade.

The first stage of a trade information display platform aggregated the commodity information of vendors in various industries so that the buyers could select the suitable commodity to buy. For example, the Alibaba Yellow Pages aggregates Chinese supplier information and display it to buyers from over 200 countries or regions worldwide through the Internet platform, thus building an online international trade negotiation and cooperation platform. The characteristics of the model in this stage are abundant and complete information, poor quality of the information, and the inability of buyers and sellers to trade online.

The second stage was an online trade platform, including B2B, B2C, and other transaction modes. It provided online trade carriers for buyers and sellers. B2B solves the dilemma of traditional bulk transactions. The participants are mainly multinational enterprises. Through online information exchange and financial payment instruments, the intermediate links are shortened, the transaction efficiency is improved, and international trade is more convenient.

The B2C cross-border retail trade participants are mainly small, medium, and micro-enterprises. It provides diversified commodities and services to consumers from different countries or regions worldwide, lowers the entry bar, saves transaction costs, opens up a new channel for small and medium-sized enterprises to sell globally, and provides consumers with a new path to buy globally. This mode, from information display to online transaction, effectively improves transaction efficiency and shortens transaction time.

The third stage is a trade industry chain comprehensive service platform, which integrates and optimizes supply chain resources, reduces intermediate links, and renders transaction services to the entire industry chain from upstream industries to downstream consumers. For example, the D.T.C. (digital trade center) model of DHgate.com integrates and optimizes industrial chain marketing, finance, logistics, and other links, provides open service ports, and creates diversified services such as trade information display online payment, financing installments, and logistics infrastructure. It charges a 5% take rate and profits from value-added information services.

At present, digital trade has entered a new stage, that is, a digital trade business operating system built on the upgrading and transforming the diversified infrastructure of global trade. It includes digital services such as merchant operating systems, super membership systems, standard product database systems, financial payments, and smart logistics. It provides a digital infrastructure for global enterprises and consumers, thereby globalizing the digital trade of "buy globally and sell globally."

Obviously, the ongoing trade digitization is not just traditional trade digitization but is led by digital trade. It covers the digitization of trade matching (offline, online, and combined digital sales, etc.); digitization of trade execution (local and cross-border logistics, warehousing, customs, licensing, taxation, etc.); digitization of trade services (market services, public services, port services, dispute resolution mechanisms, commodity inspection, finance, insurance, etc.); digitization of market entities (all trade participants, trade entities, service entities, production entities, etc.); product digitization (all finished products, semi-finished products, raw and auxiliary materials, bulk commodities, etc.); digitization of the industrial chain, including the upstream and downstream of the entire industrial chain of the manufacturing industry, industrial circulation links, and industrial capital.

The digitization of trade is believed to be the product of the integration and assistance of intelligent technology, as well as the inevitable outcome of the development of the times. The reshaping of traditional trade by digital trade is manifested in empowerment and transformation and in the use of digital technology to empower the entire trade process. As a result, the efficiency of the entire trade chain is improved. With digital technology and thinking, the digital transformation of traditional trade enterprises is accelerated. And with the new competitive advantages of trade through empowerment and transformation, traditional trading enterprises realize lower costs and higher efficiency.

Digital Trade to be Developed

Undoubtedly, in the future, the trade and taxation, customs, logistics, and other systems of various countries will be digitized and intelligentized. The data of each platform will be integrated into the workflow style. International trade will become more convenient, and trade will be more borderless. In this process, the pattern of international trade will also undergo profound changes. It is of great necessity for all countries and enterprises to seize the development window of digital trade.

From a national perspective, every state's comparative advantage is essential in determining the trade pattern. As early as the 18th century, the British economist David Ricardo pointed out that if each state could make trade decisions according to their comparative advantages, the welfare of all countries could be improved at the national level.

Compared with the UK, Portugal has lower absolute productivity in producing wine and wool textiles, but it is comparatively advantageous in making wine. Therefore, in the production of wine, the gap between Portugal and the U.K. is relatively smaller. In this case, Portugal spares no effort to produce wine while the U.K. does the same with wool textiles. In the end, when they exchange through trade, both countries can increase the total consumption of both goods.

In other words, a state's resource endowment is important in determining its comparative advantage. If a state's labor resources are relatively abundant, it will generally hold a comparative advantage in producing labor-intensive commodities. Still, if a state's capital is relatively sufficient, it is more likely to have a comparative advantage on capital-intensive commodities.

In the era of digital trade, data has become a key production factor for digital trade. Therefore, data will inevitably play an important role in determining comparative advantage and even trade structure. Countries with relatively richer data resources should export more products with higher digital content in the trade division of labor. Instead, the higher the digital content of a commodity, the higher its added value and the greater its profit margin.

Judging from China's practice, due to the large Chinese population, frequent Internet activities, and a more relaxed attitude towards privacy issues than western countries, China has many advantages in terms of the accumulation of data resources. And it is precisely for this reason that China has a great comparative advantage in many digital commodities, including artificial intelligence products. The data advantage will become a great opportunity in the background of the booming digital trade.

However, it is unavoidable that Chinese digital trading companies still face obstacles when they go overseas. In recent years, the influence of geopolitics and protectionism has expanded, and Chinese digital enterprises' overseas investment and overseas business have suffered a huge blow. In addition, China's personal information and data protection laws and regulations have not yet been perfected, especially in cross-border data flow policy and management. And the lack of international cooperation in cross-border data flow management is not conducive to enterprises going overseas.

In addition, to gain an advantage in digital trade, the most fundamental matter is the advantage of a state's digital economic strength. As for China, despite the large scale of the Chinese digital economy, it is internationalized. In the past, the development of the

Chinese digital economy has mainly benefited from the rapid growth of the domestic digital consumer market. In the digital economy fields such as e-commerce, mobile payments, social media, and search engines, some giant digital platform enterprises such as Alibaba, Tencent, and Baidu have risen.

However, compared with multinational companies such as Google, Facebook, Apple, and Amazon, the business of Chinese digital platform enterprises is mainly concentrated in the domestic market, with less overseas presence and small overseas revenue. There is a massive gap between them and American digital platform enterprises. Meanwhile, Chinese digital platform enterprises also face many barriers and challenges when going abroad.

From the perspective of system construction, though, in theory, traditional trade rules are still applicable to digital trade, and many clauses need to be revised or detailed according to specific circumstances. For example, many trades take place through the platforms, which charge corresponding service fees in the process of a trade, but there is still no legal basis for the nature of this kind of service.

In recent years, *The Cybersecurity Law of the People's Republic of China*, *The Law of the People's Republic of China Against Unfair Competition*, *The Electronic Commerce Law*, and more have been promulgated and amended one after another, providing a legal basis for digital governance and a legal guarantee for the development of digital economy and digital trade. Simultaneously, China has initially formed a digital trade management mechanism where the Propaganda Department of the Central Committee of the C.P.C., the Cyberspace Administration of China, China's Ministry of Commerce, Ministry of Industry and Information Technology of the People's Republic of China, the State Administration of Radio, Film, and Television, and the State Administration for Market Regulation collaborate. However, a systematic and perfect rule system has not yet been formed in the international governance of digital trade.

Digital trade is affecting and changing people's lives and will release greater economic potential in the future. Realizing the digital transformation of trade under the new development stage and new development pattern is an inevitable choice for the high-quality development of trade and the all-around construction of a trade power. In the next decade, digital transformation will become the main task of the governments of the major economies in the world, and international consulting agencies around digital transformation are expected to benefit handsomely from it.

2.5 The Gig Economy, a Work Revolution in the Age of Intelligence

The Internet is profoundly changing people's economic and social lives.

The rise of Internet technology and the sharing economy has increasingly blurred the boundaries of conventional working concepts, and the freelancing threshold has become lower. The labor market has transformed, and gig markets with attributes such as emergency hire, temporary hire, part-time hire, piece-rate, and "zero-hour contracts" keep emerging. More and more laborers have begun to take odd jobs through online platforms. As a result, the "Internet+ gig economy" emerged.

Meanwhile, with the rise of personalization of the modern Internet and the rise of the sharing economy model, the boundaries of the conventional working concept are increasingly blurred, and freelancing will become a critical employment pattern in the future. This background, together with the continuous impact of the COVID-19 pandemic on a global scale, further promotes the development and growth of the groups engaged in the gig economy and exhibits a trend of rapid growth trend. The era of the gig economy will come faster after the COVID-19 pandemic.

Changing

In fact, as a social phenomenon, the odd job is no recent concept. The appearance of odd jobs dates back to ancient times and has been associated with human society. Usually, people familiar with Chinese society are no strangers to freelance work, such as long-term hired hand and short-term hired hand. A long-term hired hand refers to a relatively stable work the employer offers, while a short-term hired hand is somewhat less stable.

Long and short are job stability defined by time. A short-term hired hand is usually a gig worker or a temp. And traditional odd jobs still exist in the present society. For example, southwest China provides human haulage services for consumers in need, a typical odd job with an extremely long history. Similarly, freelance writers, housekeeping services, manufacturing services (like door-to-door tailoring), etc.

It is not difficult to note that the essence of a gig is still the time a worker spends on a specific job with a specific employer using a particular ability. Certainly, as a long-existing and ancient form of work, gigs have developed with the development of factory work associated with industrialization and have been replaced by organized job positions. However, even in the heyday of industrialization, gigs persisted.

In the early stage of industrialization, some factory owners hired temporary and piece-rate workers for lower costs, which was the gig economy model during industrialization. As early as the early days of China's reform and opening up, employment groups such as gig workers, casual workers, and temps have appeared.

However, for traditional hourly workers, part-time workers, contract workers, consultants, and other gig workers, their gigs are primarily concentrated in low-income and low-skilled labor groups. Moreover, the number of traditional gig workers is scattered, the cohesion is weak, and there are not yet economies of scale. The digital age has reshaped the gig economy and ignited a work revolution.

On the one hand, compared with traditional gig labor, gig labor in the digital economy era has a strong Internet feature. The rapid development of the Internet and big data technology enables workers to get hired without labor intermediaries but directly get orders through the platforms. Workers have the autonomy to work, which means a self-employment production relationship. Meanwhile, the social contract nature of labor-capital relations has undergone a substantial change, from fixed and explicit to flexible, implicit, and market-oriented.

On the other hand, the development of new technologies such as the Internet, big data, the IoT, and artificial intelligence have tremendously transformed the current production modes of gig workers.

First, the production mode that used to be based on productive labor has increasingly turned to service labor. Second, unlike the previous gig workers who worked in fixed and centralized workplaces, gig workers of today adopt a decentralized working pattern, and their workplace has greater flexibility and autonomy. Third, traditional gig workers only need to have simple labor skills. In contrast, contemporary gig workers must be able to perform basic digital processing, and some gigs even require them to have specific professional skills. Fourth, the connection between gig workers and customers is no longer bridged by labor intermediaries but is based on the Internet platform, which adopts cloud computing to accurately match labor supply and labor demand on a large scale and with high efficiency.

In addition, contemporary gig labor is an on-demand economy, which has bred a task-oriented gig model, which requires labor suppliers to obtain labor demand information promptly and complete labor tasks "instantly." For example, online car-hailing, food delivery, errands in the same city, and other industries represent the on-demand matching of the gig economy. On-demand matching is a distinctive feature of the gig economy supported by an Internet platform or software. It makes the gig economy highly attractive to freelancers. For localized on-demand jobs, the Internet and mobile communication technology can realize instant matching of on-demand jobs, thus further promoting the development of the gig economy.

Notably, compared with the past, contemporary gigs are more flexible, and the working time and intensity depend on the workers' wishes. Without a fixed labor contract relationship between the platform and the workers, they are "free workers" in form.

The Future of Employment?

Relying on contemporary information technology, the gig economy has boomed. McKinsey & Co made a research report on future employment trends, predicting that "the future occupational trend is the gig economy" and estimated that globally, "by 2030, the annual income of the gig economy will reach US$ 1.5 trillion."

In addition, according to the *2019 China County Area Gig Economy Survey Report*, 52.27% of the population in the county market had gig income, 35.11% of the county gigs were related to the Internet, and the Internet+ gigs ranked first among various gig types. A series of trend reports has led many to believe that gigs are the "future of employment."

The gig economy appears to kill multiple birds with one stone. First, it has created a large number of job opportunities. As a new distribution form of human resources in the Internet era, it has changed the traditional single employment form and turned the original "enterprise-employee" employment contract system into a "platform-individual" transaction model, which not only saves the operation and labor costs of enterprises but also creates a great number of job opportunities.

Second, the gig economy has stimulated the vitality of innovation and entrepreneurship. Driven by the network platform, the extension of the gig economy, especially the knowledge-based gig economy, is far beyond traditional gigs' boundaries and holds greater development space and potential. In the meantime, in the Internet age, personal interests and skills can be better matched with market demand so that more practitioners' individual preferences, specialties, and resources achieve higher value, and people's "productivity" is exerted more flexibly.

Third, the gig economy makes labor more mobile. The Japanese labor market, for example, is notorious for its low mobility. And the Japanese institutional environment is most blamed. The typical features of the Japanese labor market are long-term employment, collective recruitment of fresh graduates, mandatory retirement, seniority wage systems, and vague job descriptions. These features are interrelated, and it isn't easy to adjust only one of them.

Since employees tend to stay in the same company for long, companies must set up entry and exit mechanisms. Salary systems must be based on seniority rather than competency to ensure that incentives within the same company continue to work. When an enterprise faces a new environment, it needs to adjust employment through internal job transfer. As employees continue to be transferred, the professional skills they acquire are often company-specific, which makes it difficult for them to leave the company for other jobs. More importantly, job descriptions must be vague to make them assume multiple responsibilities at the same company.

Under the influence of the COVID-19 pandemic, a major reform of Japan's employment structure might occur. Many Japanese companies are forced to work remotely, and this office model has proven effective. This will lead to a permanent shift in the way work is done. The possible outcomes of this shift to flexible work include upgrading from low mobility to a high mobility balance, more efficient resource allocation, and higher productivity.

For another example, most Chinese service enterprises adopt a fixed working hour system. Their production mechanism and personnel allocation are too rigid, and their employment flexibility is poor. With the rapid development of a new round of technological revolution and industrial transformation, service innovation has picked up the pace, and its digitization has gradually spread to all aspects of life. Consequently, the platformization of service innovation and the gig economy have taken a great leap, thereby promoting the service industry transformation.

The platform can quickly and efficiently allocate various elements by strengthening the integration of upstream and downstream resources, thus changing people's lives in all aspects of clothing, food, housing, and transportation. It provides opportunities for gig workers to realize their personal value and supports consumer demand. With the achievement of digitization, it benefits thousands of families. Meanwhile, the digital economy empowers the gig economy, increases employment flexibility, and enriches the job market.

For gig workers, flexible employment makes their fragmented time useful. They cannot only take multiple part-time jobs, but also get paid more, have more discretionary time, and are more likely to realize the exchange between talent, efficiency, and revenue, thus achieving higher value.

For employers, the gig economy can effectively solve the temporary labor demand of enterprises due to seasonality and other reasons, diversify job positions, work methods, and employment channels while minimizing labor costs and risks and improving business efficiency. Undeniably, it has created new development opportunities and holds positive significance for creating jobs, revitalizing the micro-economy, reducing enterprise costs, increasing worker's income, and promoting the transformation of the service industry.

Impacts on the Employment Paradigm

As the Internet's influence on life and work deepens, the flexible, free, and diversified online work pattern has profoundly affected the generation born after 2000, who have accepted and supported it. To a large extent, the future development potential of the gig economy has been widely recognized by society, and "gig for all" has become a trend. But in the meantime, the gig economy is not as perfect as it seems. Its work pattern breaks the traditional hiring model and brings impacts and challenges to workers, enterprises, and governments.

For workers, the biggest challenge from the gig economy is the protection of their rights and interests, the first problem being the unclear legal nexus. For example, the judgment framework of China's existing labor legal system is that the legal nexus between the laborer and the employer is based on the two classifications of labor relations and service relations. However, the verdicts given by the courts in different cases concerning the gig economy are inconsistent, which makes the identification of legal nexus ambiguous. However, the difficulty in identifying their status will prevent workers from getting the social security they deserve.

In addition, the gig economy is likely to trigger the Matthew effect (the "rich get richer, the poor get poorer" phenomenon) in the labor group. With the development of the Internet economy and digital economy, full-time working groups with a higher education background and stable income will also make better use of the gig economy platform to convert their spare time, ability, and energy into labor value, thereby increasing their extra income.

These labor groups usually possess professional skills, professional knowledge, or rich experience instead of the low income, low ability, and low education background in the traditional gig economy. They have a significant advantage in the gig economy. Groups with higher incomes or better family backgrounds likely utilize the gig economy platform to crowd out the labor groups with low incomes, low abilities, and low educational backgrounds. As the gig economy develops, the Matthew effect will strengthen the labor groups.

For enterprises, the gig economy will cause human resource management problems. In contrast to traditional enterprise organizations, the employment by enterprises in the gig economy is primarily temporary and short-term. All gig workers come from diversified sources outside the enterprise. They lack a sense of belonging and loyalty to the enterprise, making it difficult to manage them. How to effectively manage such groups will become a predicament in the human resource management of enterprises.

Usually, gig workers are mainly released and recruited by the platform, and there is a high risk of the identity information and skill level of labor groups during their review. In addition, the entry threshold for gig workers is not high, and it is easier for the identities and abilities of gig workers to fail to match the enterprise's job description and requirements, which increases the management problems of recruiting and screening them. Moreover, companies also find it challenging to manage gig workers in terms of performance appraisal, work incentives, etc.

Though the gig economy can increase G.D.P., improve employment, and promote economic transformation for the government, it comes with challenges. In addition to the difficulty in determining the status of gig workers, social security is still deficient.

At present, China implements a three-in-one guarantee mode in which the government, enterprises, and individuals jointly bear the guarantee funds. It has combined social pooling and personal accounts according to China's national conditions. However, for the workers in the gig economy, there is no related party to the enterprise, only the individual worker and the government, and the social security in the labor relationship is not compulsory, which puts the Chinese gig worker's social security issue in urgent need of legal and policy responses.

Today's gig economy is more deeply embedded in an individualized society. Supported and dominated by digital platforms, it is an ancient form of work that has been rejuvenated. It seems more like a social movement of social ethics. The gig economy is an ancient and innovative proposition requiring more social support and supervision than ever. With the gradual arrival of the metaverse era driven by technology, a "timeless, borderless" society of virtual reality is taking shape. The liberalization of work will be widely accepted in the next decade, and gigs will no longer imply precarious work but a new way of working.

2.6 The Sharing Economy Breeds a New Economic Paradigm

The sharing economy, born under the background of the Internet, as a new economic mode derived from practice, has quickly evolved into a wide social practice in the U.S., Europe, and other countries with advanced information technology, as soon as the concept of sharing is agreed upon. The sharing economy is booming from the current shared bicycles and shared cars to shared power banks and shared homestays, showing strong development momentum and potential.

As Jeremy Rifkin pointed out in his book *The Zero Marginal Cost Society: The Internet of Things, the Collaborative Commons, and the Eclipse of Capitalism*, this shared economic paradigm will go hand in hand with the past capitalist and socialist exchange economies for a long time. Inevitably, the transformation of technology and infrastructure will further reshape the system of the market economy. People will move toward a whole new economic position that transcends the market.

Indeed, the development of the sharing economy will not be smooth sailing. After human civilization went through the Bronze Age, the Age of Steam, the Age of Electricity, and the Information Age, and is once again facing a new age of sharing, how to demolish the barriers of solidified interests to the greatest extent, activate market entities to the greatest extent, and liberate and develop the productivity led by technological innovation has become a new challenge for people.

The Inevitability

In the 15th century, the advent of capitalism brought all aspects of human life into the economic realm, allowing all the items produced by people's society to be exchanged in the market as commodities. Almost all everyday needs were subsumed into capitalism, including food, drinking water, handicrafts, social relations, and even time. After that, human civilization was stamped with commercialization, and the market has defined us.

Today, however, the time of capitalism is passing, while the paradox of capitalism stands out. The inherent vigor of a competitive market has lowered the cost of running a business so much that many goods and services have become almost free, abundant, and no longer subject to the forces of supply and demand in the market. While economists will always take pleasure in reducing marginal costs, they never foresaw that a technological revolution might bring those costs to near zero.

The Fourth Industrial Revolution centered on the deep integration of networking, informatization, and intelligence is reshaping people's production and life. A great number of new scientific and technological achievements represented by mobile Internet, third-party payments, big data, cloud computing, and other technologies have entered people's daily production and life, profoundly affecting their thought, culture, life, and foreign exchange patterns first, and then politics and economics, science and technology, diplomacy, society, etc.

Over the past few years, countless consumers have begun to transform into Internet prosumers (an individual who both consumes and produces, a portmanteau of the words producer and consumer). They make and share music, videos, news, and knowledge online for nearly free, thus cutting the revenue of the music and publishing industries. Now, the phenomenon of zero marginal cost can be seen everywhere, from software and electronic goods in virtual space to physical goods in the real world.

For example, in 1999, Napster developed a platform that allowed millions of people to share music without paying producers and artists a cent. It hit the music industry hard. Next, something similar happened to the newspaper and book publishing industries. Consumers began to share their information and entertainment content through video, audio, and texts. Moreover, they completely bypassed the traditional market in a way that cost no money.

The dramatic drop in marginal costs has also reshaped the energy, manufacturing, and education industries. While the fixed costs of solar and wind technologies are high, the cost to obtain per unit of energy is low. Thousands of hobbyists are already making their own products using 3D printers, open-source software, and recycled materials at near-zero marginal cost. More and more students can attend large, free online open courses, whose marginal cost of content release is almost zero.

Meanwhile, from the Internet to the IoT, the latter's attribute of connecting everything has triggered the data explosion of a new era. Though from the perspective of the connected objects, the IoT only adds various things, it has cast an incredibly profound influence on the expansion and sublimation of the connotation of connection. It no longer takes people as a single connection center, but things can be connected autonomously without manual control.

In the IoT environment, on the one hand, everything is an entrance. In addition to the data generated by the user's active interaction, many passive data of the user will be recorded in real-time and noninductively. Therefore, enterprises can comprehensively, three-dimensionally, and dynamically understand user needs. On the other hand, smart factories in the IoT era can quickly meet users' continuously iterative customization needs through flexible production lines and transparent supply chains.

The multi-dimensional data-driven IoT can accurately grasp the demand side so that things can be directly interconnected without relying on people as the center of connection. Therefore, the IoT era's sharing platform can grasp each item's usage status in time through direct contact with the item. As long as there are good means of commercialization, all things can achieve an optimal real-time allocation of resources.

This suggests that supply and demand between people and things will become more predictable, and the prediction will be accurate. Supply, production, warehousing, delivery, etc., can be effectively and accurately calculated and supplied as per the user's big data in advance, which will eliminate material waste and incorrect distribution to the greatest extent.

Therefore, on the one hand, ample profit margins are the key to continued growth in capitalist markets, but the number of consumers willing to pay for extra fine-quality goods and services is limited. On the other hand, the IoT makes people gradually discover that physical items can be obtained on demand without owning them and that the right to use items will replace ownership. Therefore, sharing green energy and a series of essential goods and services near-free through collaborative sharing has become the most eco-beneficial development model and the best sustainable economic development model.

Under Development

As an economic revolution, the sharing economy has undergone quite a long evolution from its emergence to its development. Using without possessing is the most concise explanation of the sharing economy, but it is far from the whole picture. In fact, sharing is no new concept. Sharing is ubiquitous in the process of social and economic development. It has become a universal social phenomenon and runs through all historical stages of social development in different forms.

The sharing of information between friends and acquaintances in traditional society or the mutual lending of goods is the earliest type of sharing. Subject to the limitation of space, the objects or information shared in traditional society are usually within the scope of individuals and their abilities. The completion of sharing requires mutual trust among all parties involved, most of the shared contents are physical items, and the sharing process does not generate rewards and profits.

Since the beginning of the 21st century, with the rapid development of Internet technology, the amount of information passing through the Internet has skyrocketed. Every user can obtain information shared by strangers or share it with others through the Internet. At this stage, most of the shared objects are information, the amount of information shared has been dramatically increased, and the shared objects have begun to be stranger-oriented.

Thanks to the development of the network, information sharing is no longer limited by space constraints. Instead, the scope of sharing has been greatly expanded, but sharing information is mostly free, and there is little physical delivery. Since 2008, with the rapid development of mobile internet technology, a series of physical sharing platforms such as Uber, Airbnb, Didi, Xiaozhu, and more have begun to appear one after another. It was a substantial step that the sharing economy has finally taken from concept to reality.

Through the credit guarantee provided by the third-party platform, idle products can finally be turned into services and shared with strangers, and their suppliers will profit through such sharing. At last, sharing has evolved from purely unpaid information sharing to a shared business model of obtaining a particular reward, temporarily transferring the right to use personal items to strangers, or rendering personal services, thus completing the transformation from sharing to a sharing economy.

From the perspective of industry coverage, the sharing economy is accelerating its penetration into many areas of clothing, food, housing, and transportation, thus profoundly changing the way people produce and consume. Currently, it covers education, goods, health, food, logistics and warehousing, services, transportation, infrastructure, space, urban construction, finance, etc.

Ownership is no longer regarded as the best way to acquire a product. People no longer focus on buying or possessing a product or service but adopt a cooperative and shared mindset. They prefer to temporarily acquire a product or service or share it with others. The subjects participating in sharing are no longer just individuals, and there is a trend of enterprise-level sharing. The sharing economy's repair and remodeling of the national economy have greatly exceeded public expectations.

In 2020, the COVID-19 pandemic struck the world. The international situation was grim and complex, while China's domestic reform, development, and stability tasks were arduous. Under such highly unfavorable circumstances, new business forms and new models represented by the sharing economy have shown remarkable resilience and development potential. They have played an essential role in ensuring the supply of people's livelihoods, promoting the resumption of work and production, expanding consumption, and boosting domestic demand.

In February 2022, the State Information Center officially released the *China Sharing Economy Development Report (2021)*. Preliminarily, it estimates that the transaction scale of the Chinese sharing economy market in 2020 was about RMB 3,377.3 billion, with a year-on-year increase of about 2.9%. From the perspective of market structure, the three areas of life services, production capacity, and knowledge and skills ranked as the top three in terms of the market size of the sharing economy, with RMB 1,617.5 billion, RMB 1,084.8 billion, and RMB 401 billion respectively.

Compared to the 10% growth before, the overall growth rate is dropping. From the perspective of financing, an important development driver, the direct financing scale in the sharing economy in 2020 was about RMB 118.5 billion, with a substantial year-on-year increase of 66%. The sharing economy has bred a new production mode, consumption mode, and enterprise operation mode, becoming a future nonnegligible trend for global economic development.

The Unwalked Road

Despite the sharing economy's excellent development potential, problems come with the development of the sharing economy.

Primarily, the sharing economy is characterized by being cross-region, cross-industry and networked, and the existing legal provisions can no longer adapt to its development. As a new business model, it challenges existing laws and regulations. It is urgent that regulatory authorities improve and innovate regulatory patterns and promptly study and formulate a legal system that can adapt to the sharing economy.

Some of the regulatory terms and rules are the product of administrative regulations during the planned economy period, and do not encourage enterprises and market innovation. Moreover, some innovative enterprises are faced with unreasonable requirements from the existing system. Per the current regulations, most sharing economy enterprises are suspected of regulation violations, thus vulnerable to administrative penalties or suspension at any time. Outdated laws and regulations can no longer promote the healthy and orderly operation of the market through reasonable supervision but have become an obstacle to market innovation.

In addition, the absence of supervision and the low entry threshold of third-party platforms have made some platforms' inspection of the user qualifications not strict enough, and there are certain security loopholes in transactions. When the interests of consumers are violated, there is a lack of protection provided by all parties. Sharing platforms usually do not safeguard users against risks and accidents during the service process. So, clarifying responsibilities with existing laws and regulations is difficult.

Second, the sharing economy still lacks a sustainable business model. Currently, most products or services in the sharing economy still have no transparent business model, so it is challenging to explore specific market segments in-depth, and customer stickiness is weak. To a large extent, this drags enterprises into low-level price wars and subsidy wars, and the industry becomes wild.

In addition, the development of the sharing economy faces a common problem: the idle resources involved are a sunk cost to the owner, and there is sunk cost in the commercial operations of the sharing economy itself. It is a kind of input of the network platform for market development. Unlike the sunk cost of idle resources, this is an additional sunk cost. If this problem is not properly addressed, companies advertising the sharing economy model may go bankrupt.

At last, the proper protection mechanism and supervision mechanism of the sharing economy industry are imperfect. The government and the industry have not yet set up a regulatory system for information disclosure, competition rules, and standardized management in the sharing economy. Consumers have little trust in the sharing economy, which reduces market participation and causes the development of the sharing economy to lose the sharing mass base.

Specifically, the sharing economy uses the Internet platform to match demand and supply on a global scale in real-time. It holds excellent potential macroeconomic benefits. However, because it avoids governmental, environmental, labor, and society supervision to a certain extent, it is expected to cause many troubles. The sharing economy platforms of Airbnb and Uber have been accused of tax avoidance and violation of laborers' rights.

The 21st century is destined to be a transformative era far greater than the 20th. From the transformation of technology and infrastructure, that is, the IoT revolution ignited by the integration of communication internet, gradually maturing energy Internet, and logistics Internet, to the institutional paradox of the market economy under the technological revolution—competition and innovation drive the continuous improvement of production efficiency and the continuous decline of marginal costs. The era of sharing is quickly approaching.

In the sharing economy, where everyone creates and shares, everyone is both a co-creator and a beneficiary. The boundary between manufacturer and consumer in the past will gradually disappear, while prosumer will become more common. This shared economic paradigm will continue to go hand in hand with the past capitalist and socialist exchange economies for a long time. With the help of Internet technology, the sharing economy model will become the mainstream of business model changes in the next few decades. Whether in the field of physical entity trade or the field of virtual online games, the sharing economy model, with the help of blockchain credit technology, will be a lifestyle to build an economical planet.

CHAPTER 3

Re-upgrade of International Competition and Cooperation

IN THE PAST, NATIONAL COMPETITIVENESS MOSTLY REFERRED TO A COUNTRY'S ability to create added value in the economic sphere and its derivative areas. With the improvement of informatization, adaptability and innovation play an essential role in national competitiveness. Without informatization, there will be no modernization. As global information technology enters a new stage of comprehensive penetration, accelerated innovation, and leading development, when digital technology is increasingly infiltrating the economy and society, future national competitiveness will be more and more manifested in the ability to configure and utilize digital technology.

Whether it is the change in the influence of artificial intelligence (A.I.) on great powers, the evolution of national security governance because of the transformation of modern weapons, or the fact that quantum technology moving from theory to reality makes it possible to transform future technology, modern science and technology have profoundly changed the competition between great powers. Digital technology has given a new connotation to national competitiveness and has day by day become a more critical part of international competitiveness. It injects strong momentum into the growth of national competitiveness and is the core competitiveness of the future.

Undoubtedly, the waxing and waning of scientific and technological competitiveness dramatically affect the change of strength among countries, and the redistribution of global power in the future has quietly commenced. How to build the competitiveness of a great power and obtain the biggest development dividend in the digital age has become an important goal for all countries to seize the high ground of digital development.

3.1 Artificial Intelligence Technology Determines the Influence of Great Powers

In the late 20th century, with the development of information technology represented by A.I., the tools for human society to transform nature began to go through revolutionary changes. And the most critical sign of the transformation is that digital technology makes instruments of labor intelligent.

Intelligent tools have become typical means of production in the information society. They collect, transmit, process, and execute message data and other objects of labor. While the instruments of labor of the industrial society effectively extend human limbs, the combination of instruments of labor and objects of labor in the information society breaks the limitations of the human brain. It is a revolution to enhance and expand the functions of human intelligence and liberate it.

Today, A.I. has become an essential driving force for a new round of scientific and technological revolution and industrial transformation, and the breadth and depth of its role are comparable to that of past industrial revolutions. As the commanding height of the present scientific and technological revolution, it widely connects knowledge and technical capabilities in various fields in an intelligent manner releases the great energy accumulated by the scientific and technological revolution and industrial transformation, and becomes the center of the global scientific and technological war.

Artificial Intelligence Leads Technological Transformation

As early as September 2017, Russian President Vladimir Putin publicly stated that A.I. is the future of all mankind. It creates great opportunities, but unpredictable threats lurk there. Whoever takes the lead in A.I. will rule the world. Politically, A.I. can produce, sift, push, and block the relevant information and feed information pertinent to the society around the political demands of the ruler, thus exercising highly targeted information management and control.

Advances in A.I. are critical to the future. Economically, A.I. has become an important engine that drives economic growth.

The Industrial Revolution brought unprecedented changes to humanity. In terms of labor productivity, productivity per worker has grown tenfold in the past two hundred years. In the nearly three thousand years before this, labor productivity had hardly changed. The Industrial Revolution replaced manual labor with energy and machinery. After the Industrial Revolution, humans no longer rely on physical strength to transform the world but on skills, and human resources have undergone tremendous changes. About 90% of the workforce in modern society is engaged in skilled labor. Whether it is drivers, cooks, or service personnel, all rely on skills to work.

However, as the intelligent revolution of A.I. continues to deepen, A.I. is expected to replace almost all skilled labor with innovation. In the era of A.I., innovative talents who create new products, services, or business models will dominate the market. In the next 15 years, A.I. and automation technology will take over 40–50% of jobs, thus improving efficiency. For example, in the field of industrial manufacturing, A.I. technology will deeply empower industrial machines and significantly improve production efficiency and quality. The application of A.I. visual inspection to identify workpiece defects instead of employing workers includes the following advantages: micron-level inspection precision based on image digitization; zero emotional impact and long stable work; millisecond-level inspection speed.

The artificial-intelligence-empowered industry will accelerate the development in all walks of life and enable the economic scale to continue to expand. On the one hand, A.I. drives the intelligent transformation of the industry. Based on digitization and networking, it reshapes the production organization mode, optimizes the industrial structure, promotes the intelligent transformation of traditional fields, leads the industry to the high end of the value chain, and comprehensively improves the quality and benefits of economic development.

In terms of the military, A.I. is mainly applied to weapon systems, logistics support systems, and command and decision-making systems. It promotes tactical changes and soldier transformation, thus widely used in cyber warfare. The R&D and deployment of A.I. in the military will significantly improve the military strength of the host country and affect the international military power balance.

First, when combined with weapon systems, A.I. becomes A.I. weapons, whose most significant feature, different from traditional weapons, is the possession of intelligence or autonomy. Therefore, they are also called autonomous weapons or autonomous weapon systems and are considered the third revolution in human warfare after gunpowder and nuclear weapons.

Second, A.I. can generate a comprehensive view of the battlefield based on massive logistics support data, conduct a systematic and comprehensive analysis and evaluation of various logistics support schemes, and select the best support scheme. It is used to aid commanding and decision-making and can make critical contributions to intelligence, surveillance, and reconnaissance (I.S.R.) and analysis systems. It can restore battlefield information more completely, simulate the dispositions of forces and combat capabilities of both sides, and complete relatively accurate battlefield sand table deductions.

Third, A.I. can be applied to coordinated operations between weapons, humans, and machines to enrich tactics. In addition to traditional battlefields, A.I. used in cyber warfare has become a new type of weapon in modern warfare. In 2019, for example, I.B.M. introduced a new malware that exploits the properties of neural networks to target countries and organizations with vast computing and intelligence resources.

In acquiring global political power, the impact of A.I. on various countries' international political power is mainly manifested in the differences in their ability to obtain considerable data resources and analyze them. Today, the value of data is increasingly prominent. As a winning weapon, data has increasingly become a strategic resource for state power.

The Internet of Everything has detonated a big explosion of data. Collecting and processing this data will drive the rise and development of a number of emerging tech companies and ultimately affect the development of the world economy and military. And there is no doubt that A.I. will play an essential role in data mining and analysis.

As A.I. advances, the discussion about it is no longer limited to the perspective of science and technology. Presently, the world's major developed countries regard the development of A.I. as the primary means to enhance national competitiveness. They strive to seize the dominant right in the new round of international scientific and technological competition and strengthen deployment around basic R&D, resource opening, talent training, corporate cooperation, etc. A.I. is not only the technological label of today but the maker of today through the technological transformation it leads.

Seize the High Ground of Artificial Intelligence

Throughout history, the coupling and interaction of every technological, industrial, and military revolution have profoundly affected and even reshaped the global competition pattern. A.I. matters greatly to every country's economic strength, military strength, data analysis capabilities, etc. It is related to whether a country can gain a competitive advantage in a new round of international games and promotes changes in the international system structure.

Judging from the published national strategic plan for A.I. around the world, North America, East Asia, and Western Europe have become the most active regions for A.I. Developed countries like the U.S. have first-mover advantages in the fundamental theory of A.I., technology accumulation, talent pool, and industrial foundations, thus taking the lead in the game. Economies such as the U.S., the E.U., the U.K., and Japan have already begun to invest more in cutting-edge fields such as robotics and brain science. They have successfully released autonomous systems R&D plans such as national robotics, the human brain, and auto-piloting plans. To ensure its leading position, the U.S. published its national *AI R&D Strategic Plan* in 2016. Japan, Canada, and the U.A.E. followed closely, including A.I. into national strategies in 2017. The EU, France, the UK, Germany, South

117

Korea, and Vietnam successfully announced A.I. strategies in 2018. Denmark and Spain did the same in 2019. Various countries are leading the innovation and development of A.I. with strategies, from a scientific research model based on spontaneous and decentralized free exploration to an innovation model with national strategic promotion and guidance and thematic industrialization and application.

From the perspective of overall development, different countries around the world have placed different emphasis on the development of A.I. The development of A.I. in the U.S. is guided by military applications and drives the development of the scientific and technological industry. In terms of development, guided by the market and demand, it is focused on leading global economic development through high-tech innovation and the formulation of product standards. The development of A.I. in Europe attaches importance to the scientific and technological R&D and innovation environment and the formulation of ethical and legal rules. The development of A.I. in Asia, driven by sector application demand, concentrates on industrial scale and the R&D of vital local technologies.

Currently, China and the U.S. take the lead in the entry and layout of global A.I. They are the first echelon of the development of the global A.I. industry. In 2019, the Data Innovation Center of the Information Technology and Innovation Foundation released a 100-page research report, *Who Is Winning the A.I. Race: China, the E.U. or the United States?*, which compares the current state of A.I. development in China, the U.S., and Europe—the U.S. leads with 44.2 points, China comes second with 32.3 points, and the E.U. ranks third with 23.5 points. The leadership of the U.S. in A.I. is unquestionably evident, and China is catching up fast.

That the U.S. can occupy the leading global position in A.I. is closely related to the development of A.I. there. In 1956, A.I. was officially born in the U.S., and Carnegie Mellon University, M.I.T., and I.B.M. became its first three core A.I. research institutions.

From the 1960s to the early 1990s, AI-related programming languages and expert systems in the U.S. achieved major progress, and so has their productization. For example, in 1983, the world's first company to mass-produce computers with uniform specifications was founded. Moreover, the U.S. began to try to apply the research findings of A.I. For example, the mineral exploration expert system PROSPECTOR was employed to discover a mineral deposit in Washington.

At the same time, A.I. had just entered the embryonic stage in China. In 1978, the Science Conference in China was held in Beijing, which liberated the minds of scientific undertakings and laid a foundation for developing the Chinese A.I. industry. The same year, intelligent simulation was included in the national research plan, and the Chinese A.I. industry marched forward under the official national-level promotion.

In terms of A.I. research findings, the U.S. leads the world. According to the search results of Scopus, the world's largest citation database, in 2018, a total of 16,233 peer-reviewed papers related to A.I. were published in the U.S. The rapid growth in the number of papers mainly occurred in 2013. Though the number of such papers in China and the E.U. witnessed a similar surge during the same period, and the number of articles they published each year far exceeded that of the U.S., the quality of such papers in the U.S. was much higher than that of other regions. In 2018, the U.S. averaged 2.23 citations per paper, while the number was 1.36 in China. The U.S. also had 40% more citations per author than the global average.

Regarding critical technologies, the research findings of the U.S. remain in a leading position in the world. For example, in computer vision, the Noisy Student method developed by Google and Carnegie Mellon University has a Top-1 accuracy rate of 88.4% in classifying images, which was 35% higher than six years ago. The time required to train a large image classification system on cloud infrastructure has been reduced from three hours in 2017 to 88 seconds in 2019, and the training cost has dropped from US$ 1,112 to US$ 12.6.

From the perspective of industrial development, according to the *Global A.I. Industry Data Report (2019 Q1)* by the Data Research Center of the China Academy of Information and Communications Technology, as of the end of March 2019, there were 5,386 active A.I. companies in the world, of which 2,169 were in the U.S. alone, far more than other countries. And 1,189 were located in mainland China and 404 in the U.K., ranking third.

From the historical statistics of enterprises, the development of A.I. enterprises in the U.S. started five years earlier than that in China. They first sprouted in 1991, entered the development period in 1998, increased after 2005, and stabilized after 2013. Chinese

A.I. enterprises were born in 1996, entered a development period in 2003, and stabilized after the peak in 2015.

U.S. enterprises come out strong in patents and dominant A.I. acquisitions. For example, out of 15 machine learning subcategories, Microsoft and I.B.M. applied for more patents than any other entity in eight subcategories, including supervised learning and reinforcement learning. U.S. enterprises lead patent applications in 12 of 20 fields, including agriculture (Deere & Co.), security (I.B.M.), personal devices, computers, and man-machine interaction (Microsoft).

The talent pool is another key reason that keeps the U.S. ahead in A.I. The competition in the A.I. industry is about talent and knowledge reserves. Only by investing more researchers and continuously strengthening basic research will more intelligent technologies be invented.

The greater attention U.S. researchers pay to basic research has built the country's solid A.I. talent training system. Therefore, it has obvious advantages of research talent. Specifically, the U.S. has formed a long-leading pattern in crucial links such as basic discipline construction, patents, paper publication, high-end R&D talent, venture capital, and leading enterprises. According to MacroPolo think tank, 59% of the top A.I. research talents identified in its report work in the U.S. and 11% in China. The former is over five times the latter. And the rest of the A.I. talents are distributed in Europe, Canada, and the U.K. The talent gap is obvious.

Despite America's first-mover advantage in research findings and talent reserves in A.I., China, as a rising star, is catching up under the guidance of policies and a relaxed application environment.

Oxford Insights compared the readiness of governments for A.I., ranking the U.S. government fourth in the world after Singapore, the U.K., and Germany. But it ranks at the top of the world in critical indicators such as innovation capability, data availability, government A.I., workforce skills, number of startups, digital public services, and government effectiveness.

Though China ranks 20th on this chart, it is believed that its most significant shortcoming is the backwardness of basic research, while its comparative advantages are that the Chinese government attaches great importance to high-tech development, there is abundant data, the regulations are looser, and the number of engineers is surging. But it is visible that after years of accumulation, China has achieved a series of important achievements in A.I., forming its own unique developmental advantages. Whether it is the top-level design, the investment of R&D resources, or the development of the A.I. industry, there is a trend of catching up faster. In some core A.I. technology fields, it is already on a par with the U.S. Though it will take time to see who wins, China has become America's most feared competitor.

A 2019 report by the Congressional Research Service made it abundantly clear that potential international competitors in the A.I. market are putting pressure on the U.S., forcing it to compete in innovative applications of military A.I., and China has so far been its most ambitious competitor in the international A.I. market.

PricewaterhouseCoopers has also reported that in the era of A.I., no other country could catch up with the U.S. or China in terms of technological development or national strength, and neither the U.S. nor China could monopolize A.I. or coerce the other. The U.S. and China will account for 70% of the US$ 15.7 trillion in wealth that A.I. will bring to the global economy by 2030. The unique advantages of the two countries in A.I. will drive their development, and it will be difficult for other countries to do the same. These advantages include world-class research expertise, sufficient funding pools, rich data, a supportive policy environment, and a competitive innovation ecosystem. About half of the enterprises involved in A.I. in the world now operate in the U.S., and one-third in China.

Regarding top-level design, China and the U.S. attach almost the same level of importance. The American and Chinese governments both have elevated the development of A.I. to a national strategy, set forth a developmental strategy, and given impetus to the overall A.I. development from the national strategic level.

As early as October 2016, the Barack Obama administration released two important documents related to the development of A.I., namely *The National Artificial Intelligence Research and Development Strategic Plan* and *Preparing for Future Artificial Intelligence*. The Chinese government also included A.I. in the national government work report for the first time in March 2017. It released the New Generation of Artificial Intelligence Development Plan in July of the same year, elevating A.I. to a national strategy.

The U.S. A.I. report reflects the U.S. government's strategic orientation to maintaining its leading position in the new era. As the largest developing country, China has also made overall planning and arrangement for strategic guidance and project implementation. Moreover, both countries have established relatively complete R&D promotion mechanisms at the national level to promote the development of A.I. as a whole.

From the perspective of R&D resources input, the U.S. government's investment in R&D is relatively insufficient. Vertically, federal spending on R&D as a percentage of G.D.P. declined over the past few decades from 1.86% in 1964 to 0.7% in 2018.

At present, the annual fiscal deficit of the U.S. federal government has exceeded US$ one trillion, and the accumulated government debt is 107% of the American G.D.P. These factors will limit its long-term funding for A.I. and related basic research.

Horizontally, China and the E.U. are catching up with the U.S. regarding governmental R&D input. The U.S. share of global R&D input fell from 69% in 1960 to 28% in 2016. From 2000 to 2015, the U.S. accounted for only 19% of the growth in global R&D input, while China contributed 31%. On August 31, 2019, Shanghai announced the establishment of an A.I. industry investment fund, with RMB 10 billion invested in the first phase alone. The final scale will reach RMB 100 billion, dwarfing the input of the U.S. federal government.

From the perspective of industrial development, despite the relatively weaker overall strength of the basic layer of the Chinese A.I. industry, and a few world-leading Chinese chip companies, major enterprises are rapidly catching up, including Baidu, Alibaba, Tencent, and Huawei. They are accelerating their layout in the basic layers of software and hardware.

For the technical layer, Chinese enterprises exhibit a good momentum of development. Comprehensive enterprises such as Baidu, Alibaba, Tencent, and Huawei have arranged in core technology fields such as computer vision, natural language processing, and automatic speech recognition. At the same time, entrepreneurial unicorns are developing fast in vertical fields.

At the application level, A.I. application scenarios are diverse. Chinese A.I. enterprises have extensively deployed in fields such as education, medical care, and new retail. And a great number of A.I. enterprises compete in industries such as finance, medical care, retail, security, education, robotics, etc.

Meanwhile, compared with the U.S., China has two important advantages in developing A.I.:

On the one hand, the management system of China's A.I. ecosystem differs significantly from that of the U.S. The U.S. is a country with strong markets and a weak government. Tech companies or institutions have dominated the previous technological revolutions in the U.S., and the role of the American government in industrial development has always been limited. For China, the Chinese government plays a vital role in the economy. A top-down guided transformation is easier with strong support from national policies. The government strengthens the collaboration and resource sharing of the entire society, making it possible for China to fully occupy the commanding heights of information technology and lead in the field of A.I. technology.

On the other hand, the lower barriers to data collection and lower cost of data marking in China make it easier to create giant databases, which are essential for the operation of A.I. systems. It is estimated that, by 2020, China is expected to have 20% of the world's data share; by 2030, the percentage may exceed 30%.

In a way, the advantage of big data is also important for China to develop A.I. The development of A.I. technology requires a large amount of data accumulation for training. And China's relatively complete industrial system and huge population base give China's A.I. development an obvious advantage in data accumulation.

The advantage of the U.S. lies in the fact that it dominates the entire Western system, except for a few countries with a system that advocates domestic production. Therefore, its market, data, research scope and population are broader. However, there is a disadvantage that due to the wide range of information collection, there are inevitably different regulatory requirements in different countries. And data collection and punishment (user privacy protection) are expected to become the norm before 2035.

Great Powers Compete

In an era with no significant changes for a century, A.I., the core technology of a new round of scientific and technological revolution and industrial revolution, is of great importance to global development. A.I. technology will inevitably determine the international leadership of major powers. However, the uncertainty of A.I. development and the instability of its applications exacerbate the difficulty of technical risk management and control and bring new challenges to global governance.

First, the high productivity of A.I. means a great capability to create wealth. A.I. is obviously more advantageous to countries with the most innovative capability and an entrepreneurial economy as a high technology that leads the future. A.I. can replace manual labor with excellence, create great material wealth, and promote a country's comprehensive social governance level, economic innovation, development efficiency, national defense, security construction, etc. This means that there will be a more obvious distinction between the method and speed of wealth accumulation and the comparison of international powers. That is, the richer and stronger countries get richer and stronger, while the poorer and weaker countries get poorer and weaker. Consequently, there is an unequal distribution of wealth and injustice, which further triggers more confrontation, conflicts, and terrorism. This makes global governance more uncertain and difficult.

Second, the strong execution power of A.I. means a highly destructive power. For example, the endless emergence of new weapons and network viruses can respond quickly and tirelessly, which is beyond the human body's capabilities. Though it helps countries better perform their tasks, some forces may abuse it for a terrible purpose, thus posing a serious security threat to international society and even causing a disaster to the entire human race. Though the world may find corresponding solutions when there is an obvious crisis, the harm caused or the damage that may be caused will undoubtedly consume a lot of human, material, and financial resources, thus significantly increasing the various costs of global governance.

Finally, the high intelligence of A.I. means high political involvement. Advanced A.I. gives technology owners extra outstanding advantages. The vigorous development of

A.I., such as the industry of robots, gene sequencing, auto-piloting, smart finance, smart cities, big data processing, natural language processing, image recognition, and intelligent military systems, has changed a country's core competitiveness and economic, social, and industrial structure, thereby altering the power structure in many fields.

The power structure is a political game and a political bargaining chip. The continuous consolidation and pursuit of power is the core motivation of a country's foreign strategy and policy. In international relations, A.I. will have a significant impact directly on the subjects and objects of global governance at the field level, the institutional level, and the ideological level, thereby affecting the effectiveness of global governance.

Therefore, as major powers in the development and application of A.I. technology, China and the U.S. play an extremely important role. Both countries possess unique advantages that other countries cannot replicate. How to prevent or reduce the negative impact of A.I. technology progress on global sustainable development and strategic stability requires the full cooperation of China and the U.S.

The competition in the field of A.I. is not an absolute zero-sum game, but there is cooperative development and mutual benefit among all parties. China is relatively advanced in experimental research and application of results, while the U.S. takes the lead in basic research and cutting-edge technology exploration. There is a broad space for cooperation between the two countries. Indeed, in the development of A.I., it is not surprising that there are differences and disagreements between the two in their principled stands, interest appeals, and policy views. The key lies in rationally viewing such differences and effectively managing potential conflicts.

To this end, both China and the U.S. should think deeply and work together to have a formal conversation on the application of A.I. in the security and economic fields. They should promote the transparency of R&D of A.I., drive the rational distribution of its beneficial results on a global scale, avoid major power competition situations that could lead to catastrophic conflicts, and strive for reasonable and healthy competition and cooperation.

As Henry Kissinger put it, China and the U.S. are the countries that are most capable of influencing the progress and peace of the world in terms of technology, political experience, and history, and a cooperative way to solve the outstanding problems of both sides will be the shared responsibility of a peaceful and advancing world between them. Nonetheless, it is foreseeable that before 2035, China and the U.S. will pour huge funds into the field of A.I., compete with each other, try to win the competition with absolute advantage, and control the right of speech and dominant right of A.I. technology.

3.2 Evolution of National Security Governance

Along with the diversification of the application of science and technology, the extensiveness of the fields involved, and the pluralism of the objects of influence, while science and technology give a solid impetus for social development, it also has a series of impacts on national security governance. Among them, the changes in weapons are an important symbol of modern technological progress.

In the era of cold weapons and hot weapons, metallurgy and gunpowder based on mechanical energy and chemical energy have extended people's capability and supported them to contend for the right of way; the emergence of mechanical power has expanded the breadth of war, transforming the battlefield from two-dimensional to three-dimensional; because of the development of information technology and A.I. technology, new weapons keep emerging, thus more likely to promote national security governance and changes in the entire war mode.

The Changes in Modern Weapons

The core technologies represented by the Internet, big data, and A.I. can provide more effective maintenance and guarantee mechanisms for national security in traditional security, non-traditional security, and overlapping fields based on the practical application of evolutionary empowerment. This will fundamentally change the governance model of national security. For instance, intelligence management will rely on big data more using networks.

Military strikes will shift more from local wars in the past to the use of unmanned aerial vehicles, self-driving cars, and other facilities. With the help of satellite positioning systems, extensive data intelligence management systems, and so on, effective targeted removal is conducted; future wars will change from the past large-scale war modes that relied on human beings into one that depends on robots, intelligent facilities, and remote information control.

For example, A.I. can promote the transformation of the traditional command model into an intelligent command and control mechanism. In addition, it will also enable the extensive application of unmanned and intelligent weapons and breed new strategic combat modes such as algorithmic warfare and consciousness warfare. Certainly, the comprehensive application of A.I. also enables it to be combined with various material forces to form more effective combat capabilities in terms of situational awareness, threat analysis, strategy generation, and offense-defense confrontation.

Therefore, A.I. not only affects the form of war through purely technical aspects such as enhancing physical effectiveness, biological effectiveness, or reshaping the source of weapon energy and the principle of action, but also promotes changes in the form of war from the aspect of subject choice, such as strategic decision-making and operational command.

In addition, compared with traditional warfare, the entry threshold for information war is very low. Great powers are vulnerable to uninterrupted virtual attacks, too. Specifically, first, cyberspace surpasses the limitations of time and space, and attackers have the advantage of being unexpected; second, the anonymity and concealment of cyber-attacks enable the sponsor country of cyber-attacks to reduce the risk of being exposed, thereby making it more difficult for the attacked to identify the attacker and enabling itself to avoid more retaliation; third, it costs little to launch a cyberattack, because cyberweapons are mainly computer program codes.

In fact, the patterns and forms of modern warfare have fundamentally changed with the evolution of technology. For example, it has evolved from single-service operations of land, sea, and air to multi-service joint and coordinated operations, from tangible operations of eliminating living forces to intangible operations of confrontation in the fields of electromagnetics, networks, and cognition; from extensive operations to precise operations. The target that would require 9,000 bombs to destroy in World War II can be destroyed by a sufficiently complicated virus project in an information war. The changes in these weapons have also pushed national security governance into a whole new phase.

The Shock of Stuxnet

In December 2019, *Forbes* magazine released its list of the 12 most important new weapons of the past decade (2009–2019). It was shocking that Stuxnet, a malicious computer worm, ranked first, defeating many advanced weapons.

Stuxnet is a typical worm virus. From the perspective of transmission mode, it is mainly transmitted through a flash drive. Targeted at MS10-046 vulnerability (Lnk file {short-cut files associated with Microsoft Windows} vulnerability), MS10-061 (print service vulnerability), MS08-067 (a remote code execution vulnerability), and other vulnerabilities in Microsoft operating system, it forged digital signatures, used a complete set of intrusion transmission processes, broke through the physical limitations of industrial-specific LANs, and conducted specific attacks on Siemens' SCADA software.

From the transmission process perspective, Stuxnet first infected the external host, then the flash drive, and spread to the internal network by exploiting the shortcut file vulnerability. Next, in the intranet, through the shortcut file vulnerability, the R.P.C. remote execution vulnerability, and the printer daemon service vulnerability, it spread between the networked hosts; at last, it reached the host where the WinCC software was installed and made an attack.

In June 2010, German researchers discovered Stuxnet for the first time. Subsequently, represented by the Stuxnet operation of the U.S. against Iran, the curtain of the network virus being a super destructive weapon was lifted, and the war mode was changed.

Specifically, as a cyberweapon composed entirely of code, Stuxnet, targeted at the Siemens surveillance and data collection system used in Iran's nuclear facilities, sabotaged them by controlling the speed of centrifuge shafts. The centrifuge concentrates and purifies nuclear materials through high-speed rotation as a highly sophisticated instrument. Low-enriched uranium can be used to generate electricity, and when the purity exceeds 90%, it becomes weapons-grade nuclear material used to forge nuclear weapons.

After Stuxnet infiltrated the Iranian nuclear facilities, it first recorded information about the system's regular operation and then waited for the centrifuge to be filled with nuclear materials. After 13 days of dormancy, it released the previously recorded standard operation information to the control system. While instructing the centrifuges to run abnormally broke their maximum speed and caused their physical damage.

Therefore, after being infected with Stuxnet, thousands of centrifuges in Iran were directly damaged or exploded, resulting in the spread and contamination of the radioactive element uranium. It was a severe environmental disaster.

It was reported that Stuxnet had destroyed nearly one-fifth of Iran's centrifuges, infected more than 200,000 computers, caused physical degradation of 1,000 machines and set back Iran's nuclear program by two years. Furthermore, given the extent of the Stuxnet spread, it would be challenging to disinfect the virus in all computer equipment involved in the uranium enrichment. Perhaps these concerns led Iran to suspend uranium enrichment at Natanz in November 2010 entirely.

Symantec stated in August 2010 that 60% of the world's infected computers were in Iran. The Russian cybersecurity firm Kaspersky Labs pointed out that such a sophisticated attack can only be carried out with national support, further confirming that behind the Stuxnet attack was the U.S., Iran's arch-enemy.

During strategic deployment, the double-edged sword feature of cyberweapons is exposed. Stuxnet has exhibited shocking power beyond the control of its designers. It not only infected 45,000 networks around the world but broke into Russia's nuclear power plants. Even the computer systems of the U.S. were its victims. Today, it has become an open secret that the U.S. and Israel used Stuxnet to launch a cyber-attack on Iran code-named Operation Olympic Games. But in addition to the global impact of this open secret, it is epoch-making that the Internet virus as a weapon has become a means of confrontation between countries.

It marks the transition of cyberweapons from low-end weapons with simple structures to high-end aggressive weapons with complex structures. In fact, since Stuxnet was discovered in 2010, network experts from all over the world have been shocked by its complex structure and sophisticated design. It is more than 20 times more complicated than previous malware, exploiting multiple vulnerabilities in the operating system for automatic infection and spread. This cutting-edge weapon cost a tremendous amount of money in the development process and required a robust cyber team and engineers with knowledge of industrial control systems to work together to succeed.

In addition to the iconic transition from low-end weapons to high-end weapons, Stuxnet has shattered the fact that industrial systems closed to the outside world are safe from cyberattacks, demonstrating the great destruction of the digital Pearl Harbor cybersecurity experts have warned about for years. It operates automatically in a closed system, and once activated, it cannot be turned off until the destruction ends. Dean Turner, an expert at Symantec, stated at a congressional hearing that the threat posed by Stuxnet to the real world had been unprecedented.

Meanwhile, promoting Stuxnet to the global spread of cyber-attack technology has lowered the technical threshold for developing cyberweapons. This also means that when cyber forces of criminal groups and terrorist organizations can download the virus, modify and upgrade it, and master preliminary cyber warfare capabilities, cyber terrorism will become a severe international security challenge in post-COVID times.

With the advancement of science and technology and the frequent emergence of new weapons, human beings have entered the stage of information warfare from the stage of mechanized warfare. With the development of A.I. technology and brain-computer interface technology, the future war mode will have more possibilities. It may even break through human physiology and thinking limits and realize all-time, all-weather, all-spectrum, and all-domain combat operations.

3.3 From Looking Up at the Starry Sky to Stepping into It

At present, human civilization has approached an era of exponential growth, and human beings have a huge potential to achieve our greatest ambitions. In addition to exploring the whole world in all directions and in depth, the distant deep space is what human beings yearn for. From the moon, to Mars, to Pluto, the mysteries of the solar system are being revealed piece by piece. The vast universe is no longer as mysterious as before.

In fact, in addition to the hot new technologies such as 5G, the Internet of Things, edge computing, and AI, which are profoundly changing the world, some pioneers have been creating another world and expanding the human dimension—whether it is Richard Branson's 90-minute space trip, or the passengers signing up for Elon Musk's SpaceX program to the moon, the era of space development has begun. People have finally gone from looking up at the starry sky to stepping into it.

From the Age of Discovery to Space Exploration

Since the beginning of the Sumerian civilization, human beings have opened an era dominated by terrestrial civilization. During this period, with land as the mainstay, many empires were born—the Babylonian Empire, the Ancient Roman Empire, the Eastern Roman Empire, the Arab Empire, the Han and Tang Dynasties, the Mongolian Empire, etc. Human civilization originated on land. Though there were also famous marine civilizations in this period, such as the Aegean civilization, the terrestrial civilization was more mainstream. And the Age of Discovery had changed the world.

The opening of new routes enabled mankind to establish global connections across continents and oceans for the first time. The relative isolation between continents was broken, and the world began to connect as a whole. Since Columbus discovered the new continent, marine empires began to rise one after another, including Portugal, Spain, the Netherlands, France, etc. The birth of the U.S. is one of the fruits of Europeans' maritime activities.

The Age of Discovery completely changed the traditional social forms in South America, North America, the Caribbean, South Asia and Southeast Asia. They evolved from the ancient tribal societies to what they are today. After the Portuguese and Spaniards entered the Americas, they established their own colonies, which laid the foundation for the rise of the South American and the Caribbean countries; thirteen joint-stock companies in North America eventually founded the U.S. today through the independence movement; the British East India Company set up British India, which after independence became into the India of today.

It is the Age of Discovery that reshaped the present world. In addition to changing the global political map and state form, it also started globalization and reshaped global wealth. The demand for sails around the world created the demand for global communication, and further ignited the technological revolution and cast a profound impact on the rapid development of the present Internet prosperity, wireless communication, etc.

Though the magnificence of the Age of Discovery continues, the sea remains part of the earth, which is merely one of the eight planets in the solar system, which is merely a dot in the universe. Of the four terrestrial planets in the solar system—Mercury, Mars, Venus, and Earth, Earth is the largest. However, compared with Jupiter, Saturn, Uranus, and Neptune, it is just 1/1284 the size of Jupiter.

With this understanding, it is inevitable to explore a "new world" that is higher and farther in space. On April 12, 1961, the world's first manned spacecraft successfully took off from the Soviet Union. Soviet citizen Yuri Gagarin became the world's first cosmonaut, achieving the first human spaceflight and ushering in a new era of human exploration of space.

As the U.S. and Soviet Union contended for hegemony, on June 16, 1963, the world's first female cosmonaut Valentina Tereshkova entered space; on March 18, 1965, the Soviet cosmonaut Alexei Leonov made the first human spacewalk; on March 16, 1966, the U.S. completed the first space docking in the world's aerospace history; on July 16, 1969, the U.S. launched the Apollo 11 manned spacecraft, and astronaut Neil Armstrong was first man to set foot on the moon.

The landing of humans on the moon ended the manned spaceflight activities that were a pure parade of technical prowess. Thereafter, mankind begun to seek to establish a long-term stronghold in space—the space station.

On April 19, 1971, the Soviet Union launched the world's first manned space station Salyut 1 with the rocket Proton. By 1982, the Soviet Union had successively launched the Salyut two through five space stations and the second-generation space stations Salyut 6 and 7. On May 14, 1973, the U.S. launched a space station called Skylab with rocket Saturn V, and successively sent three batches of nine astronauts with the Apollo spacecraft.

On February 20, 1986, the Soviet Union launched the core module of the third-generation long-term crewed space station Mir. It was not finally fully completed until April 26, 1996. During its service period, it received over 100 astronauts from more than ten countries and international organizations, setting a world record of 438 days of humans living and working in space, with a cumulative service time of 748 days in space.

On September 21, 1999, China officially initiated a manned spaceflight program and determined the "three-step" development strategy. The first was the manned spacecraft program, whose main task was to launch experimental manned spacecraft and conduct space application experiments; the second was the space lab program, whose primary mission was to break through the technology of astronauts' out-of-vehicle activities, and make sure space applications have a certain scale and people to take care of within a short term; the third was the space station program, which, on the basis of the space lab, aims to ensure the space application is of large scale and with long-term care.

Regarding the manned spaceship program, on November 20, 1999, Shenzhou I made its maiden flight, achieving a major breakthrough in the round-trip between the space and the earth, which is an important milestone in China's aerospace undertaking. On January 10, 2001, Shenzhou II made its maiden flight. As China's first unmanned spacecraft, it performed a series of space science experiments to further test the coordination of the spacecraft system with other systems. In 2003, the Shenzhou V manned spacecraft succeeded for the first time in sending Chinese people to space. On October 12, 2005, Shenzhou VI took off, carrying astronauts Fei Junlong and Nie Haisheng into space, and completed the first multi-person multi-day flight test. This was a real space science experiment that people participated in, which laid the foundation for a subsequent spacewalk.

From 1999 to 2005, from Shenzhou I to Shenzhou VI, the successful launch of six spacecraft marks that China's manned space program has taken the first step, completing the preliminary supporting manned experimental spacecraft program, and laying a solid foundation for the establishment of the space lab program.

On September 25, 2008, Shenzhou VII sent three astronauts Zhai Zhigang, Liu Boming, and Jing Haipeng into space, and it was the first time that Chinese astronauts (called taikonauts) made an extravehicular walk. At the time, probably no one had thought that in over ten years, China's Chang'e spacecraft will have landed on the moon, and Tianwen (meaning "questioning the heavens" in Chinese) set foot on Mars. Since 2008, the five spacecraft from Shenzhou VII to Shenzhou XI, Tiangong-1, Tiangong-2, and Tianzhou-1 have successfully completed missions one after another, making China the third country in the world to independently master key technologies such as extra-vehicular space activity and space docking, and has accumulated valuable experience and laid a solid foundation for the construction and operation of the Chinese space station.

On June 17, 2021, Shenzhou XII successfully took off, and its three taikonauts entered the Tianhe core module. That Chinese entered their own space station for the first time meant they reached the final of the three-step development strategy.

From the Age of Discovery to the exploration of space, 60 years of manned spaceflight has built the road to space wide enough, and the dream of common people going to space is no longer that far-fetched.

A New Stage of Space Economy

While the space activities in the early days of the space age were only based on sovereign states, the boom of commercial aerospace will push the space age into another new stage —the space economy.

The space economy includes the products, services and markets created by various space activities and the related industries formed. For half a century, the space economy has undergone the construction phase of the first 20 years, whose main task was to build infrastructure, conduct preliminary applications, and gradually establish various capabilities for human exploration and development of space, and the industrialization phase of the next 20 years until today, during which expansion of application took place.

In 2008, former NASA administrator Michael Griffin delivered a speech in honor of NASA's 50th anniversary, and the concept of the space economy was born. He stated, "We were not only creating new jobs, but also creating entirely new markets and economic growth possibilities that never existed before. This is the emerging space economy, one that we do not yet understand or appreciate but will change our lives on earth."

Currently, the space economy is not an economy in space, but an economy created by space activities that benefits Earth. On the one hand, it includes various space activities and the products and services they create, such as satellite communications and television, satellite navigation and positioning, satellite weather monitoring, satellite remote sensing, etc.; on the other hand, it also involves the manufacture and launch of carrier rockets, as well as the manufacture of rockets, satellites, and ground equipment, etc.

According to the 2019 *State of the Satellite Industry Report* released by the Satellite Industry Association, the global aerospace economy reached US$ 360 billion in 2018 (US$ 348 billion in 2017). The total revenue of the satellite industry was US$ 277.4 billion, and the contribution to the global aerospace revenue from commercial aerospace accounted for 77%. Commercial aerospace has become a new driving force for the unprecedented prosperity and development of the space economy.

In this background, a great number of aerospace startups have emerged around the world. SpaceX, founded by Elon Musk, is the most innovative and productive of them all. Represented by SpaceX's Falcon rocket, major breakthroughs in low-cost carrier technology and reusable carrier technology have successfully promoted a significant reduction in space transportation costs, thus laying the foundation for the prosperity of the space economy.

In terms of space tourism, as early as 2018, SpaceX announced that Yusaku Maezawa, a Japanese billionaire and founder of Zozotown, would become the first space passenger signed by SpaceX to fly around the moon. Currently, Maezawa has paid for the entire trip, including the travel expenses of the eight crew members he sponsored. SpaceX's first passengers will begin their journey around the moon in January 2023, which will last for a week.

In February 2021, SpaceX also announced the first all-civilian mission Inspiration 4, which was carried out by the Falcon 9 carrying the Dragon capsule. According to SpaceX's official news, four passengers went into space on September 15, 2021, enjoying a three-day trip around the earth.

Though some billionaires have spent loads of money to enter space (the International Space Station) before, the number of people entering the International Space Station is extremely small and the cost is extremely high, thus difficult for popularization. However, as commercial aerospace began to render space travel services, the space age that human beings yearn for cannot wait to arrive.

In fact, in addition to Musk's SpaceX, Amazon President Jeff Bezos' Blue Origin, and Richard Branson's Virgin Atlantic are also in full swing on commercial aerospace. On the morning of July 11, 2021, local time in the U.S., Branson, the 71-year-old founder of Virgin Galactic, flew to space about 86 kilometers from the earth in the self-developed White Knight spacecraft, and returned safely to the deserts of New Mexico.

Branson not only succeeded in beating Bezos, the richest man in the world, and became the first person to travel in space, but he is also the second person over the age of 70 who went to space. In fact, Virgin Galactic lost US$ 273 million in 2021. Its business model is more closely tied to the rise of the space tourism industry than Blue Origin and SpaceX. Branson's trip to space was not only a booster for Virgin Galactic, but also a milestone moment for commercial aerospace.

In June 2021, Amazon President Bezos also announced that he and his younger brother Mark Bezos would fly into space on July 20 on a rocket developed by his own company, Blue Origin. Fellow passengers were the 82-year-old female pilot Mary Wallace "Wally" Funk, who had participated in the Mercury 13 program, and someone anonymous, who paid $28 million for the expensive ticket.

Behind the three space exploration giants of Branson, Bezos, and Musk, a new era of space economy is taking shape.

Space Activities Continue to Deepen

Once exploration activities are commercialized, the commercial institutions that support these activities are made self-sufficient, which accelerates the deepening of such exploration activities.

At present, the development of the space economy is further stimulating the innovation of cutting-edge space technology. For example, on the basis of microsatellite technology and modern communication technology, a new generation of low-orbit broadband Internet satellite constellation technology is being developed. And undoubtedly the

Starlink system of SpaceX is taking the lead.

The Starlink program was first proposed in 2015. Divided into two periods and three phases, it plans to launch a total of 12,000 satellites to multiple earth orbits between 550–1325 kilometers, so as to form a broadband satellite communication network that can cover the world. It was expected to expand the total number of satellites to 42,000 by 2019.

Since SpaceX started satellite launches in May 2019 to the present day, Starlink has completed 28 launches, and the total number of its satellites in orbit exceeds 1,000. In terms of the number of satellites it owns, SpaceX has become one of the largest satellite operators in the world.

From the perspective of the private network market, Starlink is an upgrade to operating systems like Iridium. Faced with the problems of low communication rates, expensive terminals, and expenses of Iridium and synchronous satellites, Starlink is better in terms of delays, terminal prices, traffic costs, and coverage, and can supplement the terrestrial private network at the same time. On October 27, 2020, the Starlink program sent a beta test invitation to the users who had made an appointment before, and the rates were attached to the invitation, which marked the official launch of its public satellite broadband service.

For another example, represented by SpaceX's Falcon rocket, major breakthroughs have been achieved in low-cost carrier technology and reusable carrier technology. On November 16, 2020, SpaceX's manned spacecraft Dragon was launched via the Falcon 9 launch vehicle at the Kennedy Space Center in Florida, USA, carrying three NASA astronauts and a Japanese astronaut, with the mission code Crew-1.

Crew-1 was supervised by SpaceX and the NASA. The spacecraft docked with the International Space Station about 27 hours later. The four astronauts carried out the space station mission for about half a year. This was the first approved official commercial manned space missions.

In the past, various space launch missions used to be expensive. NASA estimated that the Apollo moon landing program cost more than US$ 150 billion. From 1972 to 2011, the U.S. space shuttles have completed more than 130 missions. NASA estimated that the average cost of a single launch was around US$ 450 million, while commercial aerospace has reduced the cost of space activities through market-based competition. In 2013, SpaceX entered the commercial launch market with a price of US$ 56–62 million per launch, and the commercial launch prices of major rocket models in the world continue to decline year by year.

In addition to space exploration, space tourism, and space communication, which have taken shape now, space settlement, space mining, and space energy exploitation may further enter people's lives in the future. It is a definite fact that human society will extend and develop into space. As the great space age falls, space settlement is likely to come true.

Regarding space energy, the environment of space differs greatly from that of the earth, and the acquisition and utilization of energy will become the focus of space activities. When the space energy problem is solved, the problem of human survival on other planets will be also solved, and so will the problems of transportation and communication on other planets.

It is predicted that the opening of the space age will bring far greater changes to the human society than the Age of Discovery. Before the end of this century, human beings will have realized space immigration and space mining. Space immigration and space resources exploitation will attract more countries and commercial tech companies to explore before 2035. We will have the chance to find alternative energy sources for the earth from space, and the importance of oil will continue to be weakened. Mankind's exploration and expansion of space will transform not only the present social form, but also the current form of wealth, and more importantly, the current geopolitical model of the earth.

3.4 Quantum Science Powers the Next Technological Revolution

In 1900, Max Planck first proposed the discontinuity of energy in a paper, kicking open the door to quantum mechanics. In the quantum world, all matter can be reduced to 61 elementary particles, of which the heaviest has a mass of no more than 3.1×10^{-25} kg.

In the 1940s, Alan Turing accurately defined algorithms and described what we call a Turing machine: a single general-purpose programmable computing device that can execute any algorithm. From then on, computers have gradually developed into an industry that has profoundly changed our lives.

In 1981, famous physicist Richard Feynman, having observed the many difficulties encountered by ordinary computers based on the Turing model in simulating quantum mechanical systems, proposed the idea that classical computers simulate quantum systems. When quantum physics met computing machines, in 1985, the concept of a universal quantum computer was born. Thereafter, quantum mechanics has entered a period of rapid transformation into a true social technology, and human beings have progressed faster and faster in quantum computing application development.

At present, quantum technology has become a sharp weapon to promote the progress of the digital society. Compared with some improved technologies in the current scientific community, quantum technology has a transformative effect. It transforms the electronic computing that is occupying the mainstream position, namely, traditional and mainstream computers still use electronics as the basic carrier. Quantum technology itself, as one of the core contents of digital technology, will help the next technological revolution.

From Classical Computing to Quantum Computing

Generally, quantum computing is a new computing mode that follows the laws of quantum mechanics to control quantum information units for computing. It is completely different from the existing computing mode. To understand the concept of quantum computing, it is often compared to classical computing.

In classical computers, the basic unit of information is the bit. Everything these computers do can be broken down into patterns of 0s and 1s, and simple operations of 0s and 1s.

Similar to the way traditional computers are made of bits, quantum computers are made of quantum bits, or qubits. One qubit corresponds to one state. However, the state of a bit is a number (0 or 1), while the state of a qubit is a vector quantity. More specifically, the state of a qubit is a vector quantity in a 2D vector space called the state space.

Classical computing operates digitally using binary system, which is always in a definite state of 0 or 1. Therefore, quantum computing can realize the superposition of computing states by virtue of the superposition property of quantum mechanics, that is, not only 0 and 1, but also a superposition where 0 and 1 coexist.

While a 2-bit register in a normal computer can only store one binary number (one of 00, 01, 10, 11) at a time, a 2-qubit register in a quantum computer can hold a superposition of all 4 states simultaneously. When the number of qubits is n, a quantum processor performing one operation on n qubits is equivalent to performing 2n operations on classical bits.

In addition, coupled with the feature of quantum entanglement, quantum computers have theoretically faster processing speed and stronger processing power on some specific problems than the current classical computers that adopt the strongest algorithms.

In recent years, quantum computing technology and industry have witnessed accelerated development, and breakthroughs in quantum computing technology are mostly related to three factors: the duration that qubits can maintain their quantum states, the number of qubits connected together in a quantum system, and the grasp of what goes wrong in it.

The duration that a qubit can maintain a quantum state is called the qubit coherence time. The longer it maintains a superposition (qubits represents both 1s and 0s), the more program steps it can handle, and the more complex the computing it can perform. IBM took the lead in introducing quantum technology into practical computing systems, increasing the coherence time of qubits to 100 microseconds. When the qubit coherence time reach the millisecond level, it will be able to support a computer to solve problems that today's classical machines cannot.

Regarding the breakthrough in the number of qubits connected together in a quantum system, in October 2019, Google announced in the science journal *Nature* the use of the 54-qubit processor Sycamore, meaning the realization of quantum superiority. Specifically, Sycamore can complete the specified operation in 200 seconds, while the same amount of computation would take 10,000 years to complete on Summit, the world's largest supercomputer. It is the first time in human history that quantum superiority has been verified in an experimental environment, and *Nature* labeled it as a milestone in the history of quantum computing.

In addition to solving the problem of the number of qubits, when the qubit loses coherence, information is lost, so quantum computing technology also has to face how to control and read the qubit. Next, after the fidelity of the controlling and reading is higher, it can correct quantum errors in the quantum system.

On top of that, the researchers have drawn on the concept of error correction in classical computers to ensure that the final total equivalent quantum operation can achieve relatively high fidelity, and developed the so-called quantum error correction. Certainly, the quantum error correction at this stage still needs to break through the threshold of scale, but it is obviously no longer in the distant future.

More Possibilities

Quantum mechanics is a branch of physics that studies the behavior of subatomic particles. And quantum computers that use mysterious quantum mechanics break the limits of classical Newtonian physics. It has become a long-standing dream in the scientific communities to achieve exponential growth of computing power. Quantum computing offers tantalizing possibilities for future technological developments, and researchers who try to harness the power of this new hardware start with three types of problems.

The first type of problem involves analyzing the natural world: simulating the behavior of molecules with a quantum computer that has unmatched precision by today's computers. And computational chemistry is its largest application field. In fact, over the past couple of years, quantum computers have been making greater contribution to replacing guesswork with more and more empirical evidence.

For example, simulating a relatively basic molecule like caffeine would require a traditional computer with 10^{48} bits, which is equivalent to 10% of the number of atoms on Earth. And simulating penicillin requires 10^{86} bit—a number larger than the sum of atoms in the observable universe.

Traditional computers would never be able to handle such tasks, but in the quantum realm, such calculations are possible. In theory, a quantum computer with 160 qubits can simulate caffeine, and with 286 qubits it can simulate penicillin. This provides a more convenient means of designing new materials or finding better ways to deal with existing processes.

On August 27, 2021, Google's quantum research team announced that it had simulated the largest chemical reaction to date on a quantum computer. The related results, titled *Hartree-Fock on a Superconducting Qubit Quantum Computer*, made the cover of *Science*.

To accomplish this newest achievement, the researchers employed a Sycamore processor to simulate the isomerization of a diazene molecule consisting of two nitrogen atoms and two hydrogen atoms. At last, the quantum simulations matched those the researchers performed on classical computers, thus validating their work.

It is worth mentioning that Sycamore used in this new research is the 54-qubit processor that Nature considers a milestone in the history of quantum computing. Though this chemical reaction may be relatively simple and not impossible for a non-quantum computer to simulate, the great potential of using quantum simulations to develop new chemical substance has been demonstrated.

In addition, quantum computing is also expected to bring more benefits to AI. At present, potential applications of quantum algorithms generated for AI include quantum neural networks, natural language processing, traffic optimization, and image processing. Among them, quantum neural networks, as a research field formed by the overlapping of quantum science, information science, and cognitive science, can utilize the powerful computing power of quantum computing to improve the information processing capability of neural computing.

Regarding natural language processing, in April 2020, Cambridge Quantum Computing announced the success of a natural language processing test performed on a quantum computer. This is the first successful validation of quantum natural language processing application on a global scale. Researchers used the "eigen quantum" structure of natural language to translate sentences with grammar into quantum circuits, implement the process of program processing on quantum computers, and get answers to the questions in the sentences. With quantum computing, it is expected to achieve further breakthroughs in semantic awareness in natural language processing.

Finally, there is the possibility of quantum computing to optimize complex problems that often have too many variables for today's computers. One use of quantum computing for complex problems, for example, will build better models of financial markets. By inventing new numbers, it strengthens encryption, and improves operational efficiency in chaotic and complex areas such as transaction clearing and reconciliation. A quantum system can handle derivatives pricing, portfolio optimization, and risk management in highly complex and changing situations.

The Battle for Quantum Supremacy

At present, around the world, governments of many countries continue to set forth development strategies to support quantum information technology, and grant ample funds for its research that is mainly centered on quantum computing. The battle for quantum supremacy continues to attract attention. There is nothing political in quantum supremacy as it might suggest. Instead, it is a purely scientific idea that when a quantum computer surpasses the existing strongest classical computer in a certain problem, it holds quantum superiority, or quantum supremacy.

Based on quantum superposition, many quantum scientists believe that the computing power of a quantum computer in certain tasks will far exceed that of any classical computer. But for the moment, achieving quantum supremacy remains a protracted battle.

Fundamentally, it is because of the conditions to realize quantum supremacy. Scientists believe that quantum supremacy is possible when more than a certain number of qubits can be precisely manipulated. This contains two key points: the number of qubits manipulated, and the precision of the manipulation. Only when both conditions are met can superiority of quantum computing take place.

However, whether it is the Sycamore that has achieved quantum supremacy with 54 qubits, or the Jiuzhang quantum computing prototype that has built 76 photons to achieve it, though the number of manipulated qubits continues to rise, people still need to face the accuracy of quantum computing and the great potential of supercomputing engineering.

The duration that a qubit can maintain a quantum state is called the qubit coherence time. The longer it maintains a superposition (qubits represents both 1s and 0s), the more program steps it can handle, and the more complex the computing it can perform. When qubits lose coherence, information is lost. Therefore, quantum computing technology also has to face how to control and read the qubit. Next, after the fidelity of the controlling and reading is higher, it shall correct quantum error in the quantum system.

Meanwhile, the algorithms and hardware of classical computing continue to be optimized, so the potential of supercomputing engineering must not be underestimated. For example, I.B.M. claimed that it would take around two days for classical simulation to achieve 53-bit, 20-depth quantum random circuit sampling.

As mentioned earlier, the realization of Sycamore's quantum superiority depends on its sample size. When collecting one million samples, it has an absolute advantage over supercomputers, but to collect 10 billion samples, it only takes classical computers two days while Sycamore needs 20 days to complete such a large sample collection, which makes quantum computing lose its superiority.

In addition, for a long time, the superiority of quantum computers was limited to specific tasks. Google's quantum computer, for example, is aimed at a task called Random Circuit Sampling. Generally, when choosing this specific task, meticulous consideration is required. This task is more suitable for the existing quantum system and is difficult for classical computing to simulate.

This means that quantum computers do not outperform classical computers in all problems, but only some specific ones, for which they design efficient quantum algorithms. For problems without quantum algorithms, quantum computers have no advantage.

In fact, this is also the creative breakthrough of the Chinese team's announcement of quantum computer Jiuzhang after Sycamore to achieve quantum supremacy. Sycamore relies on its sample size to realize quantum superiority. In fact, though it takes only 200 seconds for Sycamore to collect one million samples, and two days for the supercomputer Summit to do the same, which exhibits quantum computing's superiority over supercomputers, if it is 10 billion samples to be collected, it still takes only two days for a classical computer, but 20 days for the Sycamore. Under such a condition, quantum computing loses its superiority.

However, the quantum computing superiority reflected in the Gaussian Boson Sampling

The problem, which Jiuzhang has solved, does not depend on the sample size. Meanwhile, in terms of velocity equivalent, Jiuzhang is 10 billion times faster than Sycamore on the same track. According to the current optimal classical algorithm, it takes Jiuzhang 200 seconds to collect the 5,000 samples, Sunway TaihuLight, a Chinese supercomputer, 2.5 billion years, and Fugaku, the world's number one supercomputer, 600 million years to do the same.

In addition, in terms of state space, Jiuzhang is also far superior to "Sycamore with the advantage that its output quantum state space scale reaches 1030. The outstanding performance of Jiuzhang has firmly established China's leading position internationally in quantum computing research. Also, it is a major achievement in quantum computing. The quantum supremacy of the second demonstration of Jiuzhang not only proves the principle, but also shows that Gaussian Boson Sampling may have practical applications, such as solving specialized issues in quantum chemistry and mathematics.

More broadly, mastering the ability to control photons as qubits is a prerequisite for building any large-scale quantum internet. But in general, the competition between quantum computing and classical computing will be a long-term dynamic process, regardless of the quantity and accuracy of quantum computing, and the potential or limitation of classical computing.

Some things in quantum physics seem chaotic to laymen, and some seem to make no sense at all. But this is what's fascinating about quantum mechanics, and the whole point of scientists' work. Quantum mechanics can be interpreted to mean that physicists are trying to find a certain "match" in the real world to the mathematical theory of quantum mechanics. On a deeper level, each kind of interpretation reflects a certain worldview.

In the long run, under the deployment and development of the world, quantum computing will most probably eliminate the time barrier completely, lower the cost barrier accordingly, and breed a new type of machine learning paradigm in the future. However, before a general-purpose quantum computer with general functions like traditional computers takes shape, quantum computing still requires long exploration, but quantum technology will definitely be present in the next technological revolution. Quantum science will make further major breakthroughs in this world, and new physics theories will emerge based on it. Humans will begin to explore and think about multi-dimensional space, and the time travel will change from a theoretical conception to a scientific research topic with formal experiments.

3.5 New Competition in the Chip Market

The COVID-19 pandemic has motived unprecedented efforts in the scientific community, demonstrating the inherent logic of the modernization of science and technology. After the pandemic, basic scientific research will become the core element of the industrial competitiveness of various countries because the emergence of robot-based intelligent manufacturing and flexible manufacturing has fundamentally changed the current manual labor-based manufacturing industry.

The manufacturing industry will get cheaper because of the introduction of robots, becoming the link with the least technical content and competitive advantage. Every country will assemble and produce corresponding products according to the living needs of its citizens. However, at this time, the upstream of assembly, that is, the basic materials for manufacturing components, will become the key to competition, and the pricing power of the industrial chain will undergo a major change from the current terminal commodity-centered pricing to basic materials-centered pricing.

The chip, as the soul of the market, is also one of the three elements of the information industry. The technology and business competition for chips will inevitably experience new challenges, and there will be a reshuffling in the market.

The Chip Situation

People are amazed at the magical functions of high-tech electronic products in the information age. And the core device that endows these products with magical functions is the integrated circuit chip.

The chip adopts hundreds of complex processes to interconnect the transistors required in a circuit, including diodes, resistors, capacitors, inductors, and other components, and wiring to form a circuit. Concentrated on a small piece or a few small pieces of silicon, it is packaged in a shell and becomes a miniature structure with the required circuit functions. The biggest feature of the chip is that a chip as small as a fingernail holds a huge number of electronic components. It is conceivable that the technical difficulty is exceptionally high.

In 1946, the world's first general-purpose electronic computer Eniac was born. Still, it weighed more than 30 tons, covered an area of more than 170 square meters, and was equipped with 18,000 electronic tubes, thousands of diodes, resistors, and other components. There were as many as 500,000 soldering points inside its circuit. Its surface was covered with meters, wires, and indicator lights. It's worth mentioning that it consumed over 174 kilowatt-hours of power. Every time it was used, the lights in the town would dim. To make matters worse, one tube burned out on average every 15 minutes, and scientists had to keep replacing them.

Regardless, this behemoth, which people now find peculiar, was 200,000 times faster than manual calculations at the time and 1,000 times faster than a relay computer. What contributed significantly to the operation of Eniac was the use of vacuum tubes, which performed the calculation, and the storage medium of the memory was a kind of punched card. Though this computer outperformed people greatly due to its large size and the slow information storage, people's wish to downsize the computer and improve the computing speed grew stronger and stronger.

The transistor was therefore invented: John Bardeen (1908–1991), Walter Brattain (1902–1987), and William Shockley (1910–1989) at Bell Labs in 1947 co-invented it. With this epoch-making invention, they won the 1956 Nobel Prize in Physics. The invention of the transistor unveiled the mystery of semiconductor devices, opened the development history of chips, triggered the third industrial revolution, and led human society into the electronic age.

In May 1952, British scientist G.W.A. Dummer (1909–2002) first proposed the idea of integrated circuits. In 1958, Jack Kilby (1923–2005) at Texas Instruments and Robert Noyce (1927–1990) at the Fairchild Semiconductor Corporation independently invented the integrated circuit. In 2000, the Nobel Prize in Physics was awarded to Kilby and others for their fundamental contributions to modern information technology.

In 1958, Texas Instruments displayed the world's first integrated circuit plate, marking the world's entry into the era of integrated circuits and lifting the curtain on the information revolution in the 20th century. Today, people use computers $1/n$ the size of the early behemoth. Therefore, integrated circuits have played an extraordinary role in human history, and chips have penetrated every aspect of our daily lives.

The electronic alarm clock that wakes people up in the morning, music, and LED screens are controlled by chips; when the LED desk lamp is turned on at the night table, a small chip helps stabilize the voltage; when the mobile phone is on, several chips are working at the same time; in the kitchen, the refrigerator and microwave ovens are controlled by the chip. Whether it is a small daily item, such as a TV, washing machine, mobile phone, computer, and other household consumer goods, or a giant machine, such as CNC machine tools in traditional industries, missiles, satellites, rockets, and warships in the national defense industry, chips are inseparable.

The Waxing and Waning of Chip Power

Strong chips make advanced technology. When science and technology thrive, the country thrives. The COVID-19 pandemic has profoundly demonstrated the importance of chips to a country. The infrared temperature sensor chip is the core material of badly-needed resources such as infrared temperature detectors, infrared imaging monitors, and thermometers. And the kit that uses biochip technology significantly reduces the time for virus detection. In addition, for example, on smart medical platforms, various informatization methods and techniques are also inseparable from the guarantee of communication chips. The chip industry has already become a powerful weapon for which countries contend and even an effective means to win international competitions.

Globally, due to the diversification of demand in the application market and the modularization and international division of labor in the industrial chain, the overall monopoly of the chip industry is weakening. And as the industrial layout of different countries is closely linked, their strength waxes and wanes.

The U.S. is evolving towards a comprehensive ecosystem while maintaining a first-mover advantage in the global chip industry. In 2018, chip makers with and without factories in the U.S. together occupied 52% of the entire semiconductor market. And by virtue of their pioneering status, they have formed a market with an entire industrial chain, including almost all chip categories, production equipment, and materials, thus controlling the upstream high value-added end. Moreover, giants have begun to deploy closed systems from design to application. For example, Intel acquired Israel's Mobileye to get involved in autopiloted vehicles, and terminal companies such as Google and Amazon have started independently developing chips to create a closed-loop ecosystem for their products.

Europe and Japan have opened up differentiated battlefields based on occupying the highlands of materials and equipment. Europe's strong basic R&D capabilities and traditional chip I.D.M. manufacturer models, coupled with developed mechanical engineering, provide a vast application market for automobile manufacturing, thus enabling itself to lead the design and manufacture of industrial and automotive semiconductors.

Japan avoided the mainstream cloud computing A.I. chip competition and turned to the R&D of edge computing-oriented terminal A.I. chips; Europe launched the 62-million-euro Power Semiconductor Electronics Manufacturing 4.0 program in 2016 to realize smart manufacturing with a mix of advanced manufacturing technologies.

South Korea and Taiwan focus on consolidating their positions in the industrial chain. Historically, the development of chips in South Korea and Taiwan has benefited from the second industrial transfer centered on the U.S. South Korea's government + tycoons model, which supports the vast industrial chain led by Samsung and SK Hynix.

It is a replica and continuation of the previous era in the U.S. For example, Samsung's integration of design and manufacturing has made it surpass Intel and become the world's leading chip company.

Taiwan focuses on downstream wafer foundries and close beta testing. In terms of close beta testing, Taiwanese companies like ASE Group won 54% of the global market share in 2018. The Taiwan Semiconductor Manufacturing Company (TSMC) led the mass production of the 7 nm (nm = nanometer, or one-billionth of a meter) process, won nearly 50% of the market in the second quarter of 2019, and completed the world's first 3D IC packaging.

In the third industrial transfer, mainland China has risen. From the perspective of domestic demand and export, it is the largest consumer of chips, but from the perspective of the industrial chain, it is still heavy at both ends and light in the middle. Design and close beta testing are growing rapidly, while the core manufacturing technology remains highly dependent on imports. In 2018, the revenue of China's IC design industry, represented by Huawei HiSilicon, was RMB 251.5 billion with an annual growth rate of 23%; the Chinese close beta testing swallowed 12% of the global market share, but the integrated circuit trade deficit was as high as three times.

With the emergence of a new round of technological revolution and industrial trans-formation, some critical scientific issues and key core technologies will continue to make breakthroughs. The acceleration of industrial renewal and iteration significantly impacts the global economic structure and competition pattern. After the COVID-19 pandemic, as the current pricing of terminal commodities is changed to the pricing of industries and commodities that are centered on primary materials, the global competition for chips will continue to escalate, and basic scientific research will increasingly become the core element of the industrial competitiveness of various countries.

However, the technical end of the current chip technology is approaching, and the application of physical materials will soon be brought to their extreme. However, before 2035, chip technology will mainly focus on upgrading current semiconductor technology. After 2035, chip technology will be explored at the technical level in combination with life engineering, that is, the direction of the development of human cell technology and the direction of quantum science. These are the two major expansion routes of the currently foreseeable chip technology. Certainly, it cannot be ruled out that the accelerated discovery of space exploration technology might lend us some help via dark matter mining in outer space to achieve a breakthrough in the third path of chip technology.

But it cannot be ignored that if the U.S. continues to block and suppress China in the chip industry, the Chinese chip industry is expected to achieve a major breakthrough around 2035. At that time, China will have had a complete and independent industrial system in the chip industry. All existing industrial chain shortcomings in China will have been overcome. Currently, the chip industry technology in China is not the most advanced in the world. Still, its cost must be the most advantageous for the same level of technology, which will greatly take the market share from developing countries.

3.6 The Future of Investment in Africa Has Come

The fertile soil of the African continent stores the DNA of the earliest human beings. Still, there is a considerable phased gap between Africa and the development of the contemporary world. When people's impression of Africa is still stuck in the history of African colonialism and waves of refugees, it has escaped from the ancient "poverty trap" of being underdeveloped for centuries. It has become the region with the most development potential in the world with its rich mineral resources and lower development rate.

The venture capital industry and innovation ecosystem are emerging in Africa—Africa has witnessed a steady increase in venture capital inflows over the past five years. From 2012 to 2018, investment in the African venture capital market grew at a CAGR of 46%. Every year there is more news about new peaks in funding rounds and transaction volumes about Africa or African startups—it is the right time to invest in Africa.

Though Africa attracted much less foreign direct investment in 2020 due to the COVID-19 pandemic and high resource prices, suffering its first economic recession in nearly 25 years, this does not change the fact that Africa is still an untapped investment gold mine. Whether for a country or a company, the future of investment in Africa has come.

Why Africa?

Africa, bordering Europe and Asia, holds a vast territory with a total land area of about 30.2 million square kilometers, accounting for 20.4% of the world's total land area. It is the second-largest continent in the world after Asia. The equator runs through it. Three-quarters of Africa's area is in the tropics between the Tropic of Cancer and Tropic of Capricorn. The annual average temperature in most African areas is above 20 degrees Celsius. The climate is usually warm and hot, thus the name a tropical continent.

Plateaus and deserts dominate the terrain of Africa. There are scattered basins and rift valleys and a few plains. The plateaus at an altitude of 500 to 1,000 meters account for over 60% of the entire continent. The appearance of the African continent can be described as a vast plateau that rises suddenly from the long and narrow coastal zone in the southeast and descends to the northwest until it becomes a plain near the Mediterranean Sea.

The desert area, mainly composed of the Sahara Desert in the northwest and the Namib Desert in the south, accounts for 1/3 of the total area of Africa. Central Africa is home to the largest basin in the world, the Congo Basin. The plains below 200 meters above sea level are mainly distributed in the Nile delta, the Niger delta, and the coastal areas, accounting for less than 10% of the entire continent. In addition, another prominent feature of the African terrain is the extensive rift valleys, which are widely distributed in West and East Africa.

Such terrain diversifies the African climates. The central Congo Basin and the Guinea Coast belong to the tropical rainforest climate. The Mediterranean coast, hot and dry in summer and warm and rainy in winter, has a subtropical Mediterranean climate. The Sahara Desert in North Africa and the western part of the South African Plateau, with rare rainfall, have tropical desert climates. Other vast areas are rainy in summer and dry in winter. They mostly have a savannah climate.

The regional differences in precipitation determine the distribution pattern of African water systems. The equatorial region rains all year round, so there is a good water source. And its surface is not undulating, so many rivers form the famous Congo River system. The southeastern part of the continent is affected by the warm and humid airflow from the Indian Ocean all year round, so there is abundant precipitation and sufficient surface runoff, forming larger water systems such as the Zambezi River.

In the vast arid areas, the precipitation is scarce while the evaporation is strong, so there are few rivers, and the river network density is small. African rivers are characterized by swift torrents, many shoals, and great waterfalls, thus the great prospect of hydropower. However, those are not good for water transportation.

Geographical features determine that Africa is a continent that is difficult to access from the outside and divided from the inside. On the one hand, it effectively resists the invasion of foreign enemies. Still, on the other, it also hinders communication within Africa and other regions, which is one of the causes of the backward development of African civilization.

In addition, because of the terrain, the transportation between the inland plateau and the seaside ports in Africa is challenging. The transportation problem has long been an obstacle to Africa's economic development. Moreover, due to topography and climate, there is no broad area of arable land suitable for agricultural development in Africa. There are many mosquitoes in tropical regions whose spread of infectious diseases is not conducive to the development of animal husbandry. Even today, though the situation has improved, Africa still suffers from frequent famines and has to import food in large quantities.

However, from the perspective of natural resources, Africa's proven mineral resources have advantages that are incomparable to anywhere else. There are rich reserves of oil, natural gas, iron, manganese, chromium, cobalt, nickel, vanadium, copper, lead, zinc, tin, phosphate, and more. African gold and diamonds have a long-standing reputation. Furthermore, Africa is home to various animal and plant resources. There are at least 40,000 species of plants. And on the vast grasslands live a large variety and quantity of wild animals.

For example, like a natural treasure bowl, the Democratic Republic of the Congo (D.R.C.) houses a complete range of mineral resources worth US$ 2.5 trillion. It is therefore called the world's geological museum, the world's raw material warehouse, a Central African gem, and a geological miracle. Its territory stores abundant energy minerals, metallic minerals, and non-metallic minerals, among which copper, cobalt, diamonds, tin, niobium, and tantalum occupy an important position worldwide.

The D.R.C. is also home to the most critical diamond resource in Africa. According to statistics released by the U.S. Federal Bureau of Investigation, the D.R.C. currently has about 150 million carats of diamonds. Among them, the Mbuji Mayi deposit is the largest and world-famous diamond deposit in the D.R.C. This deposit stores vast resources, but the quality of its diamonds is low, and most of them are industrial-grade diamonds.

From the perspective of resources, any foreign investment is related to them. Africa's natural resources are undoubtedly one of the reasons why it has become a gold mine for investment, but there is more to come.

Demographic Dividends Trigger Changes in Africa

Africa has become the region with the fastest-growing population in the world. From 140 million in 1900 to 1.25 billion in 2017, the African population has experienced near-explosive growth over the past four decades. Today, one in six people lives in Africa, and one in three newborns is born in Africa.

In 2017, Africa's annual population growth rate was as high as 2.7%, nearly three times the global average (1.1%) and four to five times the rate of China. By 2050, Africa's total population will reach two billion, accounting for over one-fifth of the global population.

In terms of the fertility rate, the average fertility rate in Africa (that is, the average number of children per woman within the reproductive age range) in 2017 was as high as 4.9, much higher than the global rate of 2.4 and China's 1.6. Health care in Africa has improved significantly over the past half-century, and infant survival and life expectancy have approached global averages. Such rapid population growth has had a devastating impact on the age structure of Africa's population.

Since 1980, the average fertility rate in Africa has been slowly declining due to changes in ideas and the popularization of birth control means. Such conditions have allowed Africa to enter the golden age of a demographic dividend. At this time, a country's fertility rate is rapidly declining while aging has not yet begun.

Under such circumstances, the proportion of child support is low. In contrast, the proportion of the working-age population is high, thus forming a situation of abundant labor resources, increased savings, high investment, and favorable economic development. This phenomenon, which economists call the demographic dividend, is one of the reasons for China's rapid economic growth in the past three decades and optimism about the African economy.

On the one hand, the African population is young. The average age of the African population is only 19.4 years old, far lower than the world average of 30.6. The youthful population structure of Africa is conducive to increasing the labor force and cultivating new consumption habits, thus laying a solid foundation for the development of the Internet industry and high-tech industry.

On the other hand, unlike in China or upper-middle-income countries, the labor force participation rate in Africa has been rising slowly since 1997. This is closely related to the changing cultural concepts and social customs there in the past 20 years:

- Fertility rates are declining.
- Late marriage and childbearing have become more common.
- Women's education levels continue to improve.
- More and more women are choosing to work.

As a result, a younger demographic and a steadily rising labor force participation rate gives Africa more abundant labor resources than the rest of the world. Moreover, the demographic dividend is accompanied by a sufficient and low-cost labor supply and the group effect that the younger generation will breed a huge potential Internet consumer market.

Opportunities abound in rapidly growing Africa: how to feed Africa's growing population presents huge food trade opportunities; how to improve Africans' medical and diagnostic standards presents biomedical trade opportunities; how to improve Africans' standard of living offers a significant number of trading opportunities for living materials, including the investment opportunities for new energy vehicles; how to improve the technological living standards of Africans presents a great number of Internet entrepreneurial opportunities.

As the African population peaks, Africa will bring the dividend of the era with a steep growth curve to the development and popularization of the Internet for a long time to come.

Why Does China Invest in Africa?

Though the great navigator Zheng He had reached the coast of East Africa as early as the 15th century, the exchanges between modern China and Africa began in the 1950-60s—when African countries were fighting for independence. Tanzanian President Juliet Julius Nyerere turned to China for support, hoping to unite the third world.

As international political and economic games intensify, the world is undergoing drastic changes that have not been seen in a century. Developed western economies have introduced strict investment restrictions on the grounds of national security and environmental protection. International investment protectionism continues to escalate, curbing China's outbound direct investment in developed countries. Instead, the Belt and Road Initiative countries and African countries have become a new growth pole for China's outbound investment.

With the proposal and implementation of the Belt and Road Initiative, the strategic position of African trade has become increasingly important. The new development of Sino-Africa economic and trade relations will contribute to global economic stability. For China, increasing investment in Africa is conducive to obtaining new production capacity cooperation opportunities, natural resources, and cheap labor, thus transferring Chinese marginal industries, promoting the upgrading of industrial structure, and boosting the high-quality development of the Chinese economy.

For Africa, direct investment from China can inject new funds into African economic development, help African countries alleviate both employment and poverty problems, and make the relevant planning in the U.N.'s Millennium Development Goals come true. In fact, on the global economic map, Africa has become hot and is heating up daily.

In the past decade, Africa was the fastest growing place other than China and Southeast Asia, with growth rates ranging from 4% to 6% in most years. In this process, the power of China cannot be underestimated. In 2013, a critical shift occurred in Africa. China has overtaken the U.S. as the continent's largest direct investor in foreign direct investment.

In recent years, the economic complementarity of China and Africa has gradually stood out. Africa is expected to become the engine of world economic growth in the next century. Since 2017, the direct investment of the U.S. in Africa has witnessed a net outflow year by year. China has instead begun to fill the void it left and replace it as Africa's largest investor.

It is worth mentioning that most private Chinese enterprises' investment in Africa is directly driven by the development prospects of the African market and the increasingly deeper connection with China's industrial chain and consumer market. Just as Western multinational corporations were attracted by the charm of the Chinese market 40 years ago, today's private Chinese enterprises are under the spell of an African future.

According to data from the Ministry of Commerce of China, private Chinese enterprises account for 90% of the total Chinese enterprises that invest directly in Africa and 70% of China's total direct investment in Africa. There is no doubt that Chinese state-owned enterprises (S.O.E.s) are still major investors in large-scale programs in terms of single investment volume, especially in the fields of infrastructure, energy, and resources. Due to the strategic nature and long payback period of these investments, S.O.E.s have a natural investment advantage.

Since 2010, one-third of Africa's grid and power infrastructure has been invested in and built by Chinese enterprises. Through investment by Chinese S.O.E.s, China has also become Africa's most important investment partner in energy infrastructure. However, it is worth reminding us that China's foreign direct investment in Africa needs to pay more heed to the complementary effect of China's economic development rather than copy its development model.

We see that today's African economies are in steady upward development. There is sustained economic growth, an explosion of demographic dividends, and a gradual market opening in Africa. As a third-world country, Africa continues to narrow the distance from the developed world, and the Internet serves as a catalyst to accelerate this process. Be it countries or companies, the future of investment in Africa is coming. In addition to the Taiwan problem, the focus of the game between countries in the world before 2035 is Africa (the Asia-Pacific region will have a relatively balanced situation in international relations before 2035). Both China and Western countries led by the U.S. will pour a lot of resources and funds into Africa, trying to gain influence and right of speech in its political system, cultural education, and resource control.

It is foreseeable that until 2035, the U.S. will continue to contend with China in Africa. The U.S. will continue to create a turbulent environment in Africa through its political and military means to threaten China's investment in Africa to varying degrees. Whether it is at the economic, political, cultural, or military level, Africa will become the focus of the next game between China and the U.S. They, Russia, and other European countries all hope to gain corresponding dominance in Africa. The most important influence is the contest between China and the U.S. in Africa.

CHAPTER 4

Technology Empowers the Future Society

THE INDUSTRIAL REVOLUTION IS THE STARTING POINT OF MODERN civilization and has fundamentally changed the production mode of human beings. Industrial development has enabled human beings to have a greater ability to transform nature and obtain resources. People directly or indirectly consume its products, dramatically improving their living standards. So far, the industrial age marked by scientific rationality and technological progress has been the most brilliant stage of human development. Since the birth of industrial civilization, industry has determined the survival and development of human beings in a certain sense.

Under the long-term accumulation and nurturing of the first three industrial revolutions, the Fourth Industrial Revolution, characterized by intelligentization and represented by cutting-edge technologies such as artificial intelligence, quantum communication, biotechnology, and virtual reality, is rising faster than ever. It is another major event that has greatly changed human beings' social and economic life after the technical revolutions of steam, electricity, and information.

The core of this technological revolution is the deep integration of networking, informatization, and intelligentization. While improving productivity and enriching material supply, it also reshapes labor forms and requirements of combining human and machine power. It adds new content and approaches to the policy side to empower the world of tomorrow.

4.1 Internet of Everything reshapes the digital world

Thanks to the development of communication technology, we are embracing an unprecedented digital world.

As early as the 22nd meeting of ITU-RWP5D (Responsible for the overall radio system aspects of International Mobile Telecommunications (I.M.T.) systems) in 2015, the International Telecommunication Union (I.T.U.) elaborated on the vision of the fifth generation of mobile communication (5G):

1. Enhanced mobile broadband (eMBB)
2. Massive machine-type communication (mMTC)
3. Ultra-reliable and low latency communication (uRLLC)

Among them, eMBB, as an upgrade of the existing 2G/3G/4G technologies, requires the mobile communication rate to be increased by ten times based on 4G to support applications with higher data transmission requirements, such as VR/AR, 8K video, A.I., etc.

Collectively referred to as mobile IoT scenarios, mMTC and uRLLC are an application vision that has never been proposed before 5G and the biggest difference between the present and the past. Today, trillions of sensors are embedded in every corner of society, forming a new vision of the Internet of Everything. From the Internet to the IoT, the latter's nature of connecting everything is triggering a data explosion in recent times.

More cell phones than toilets

At present, the penetration rate of smartphones has reached unprecedented saturation. In China, for example, according to the data from the Ministry of Industry and Information Technology of China, the number of smartphones per 100 people in China has reached 112.2, indicating more than one mobile phone per person. With the advent of the 5G era, mobile phones, as the core product of the user end, will remain the world's leading consumer electronics.

In the past 40 years, from the I.B.M. personal computers from 1981 to 1992-1995, when Microsoft successively released the Windows system centered on mouse movement, and then to 2007, when the first iPhone, which was installed with a touch interface based on finger sliding, came out, the user interface system has undergone three significant evolutions. Along with that, there were all-round changes in the form of equipment: software upgrades, hardware updates, and drastic changes in the market structure. In terms of hardware, users witnessed the shift from desktop computers to laptops, feature phones, and smartphones.

The mobile phone industry has experienced the transition from feature phones to smartphones. After the iPhone, the industry has been looking for the next computing terminal of smartphones, such as smart glasses, smart watches, and so on, but they have failed to replace smartphones. Regardless of market value or frequency of use, smartphones remain the center of the user side.

Since 2019, the world has entered the 5G era, and the vision has become clearer from the era of smartphones to the era of consumer IoT centered on mobile phones, which remain the core products of the 5G era. To a certain extent, the COVID-19 pandemic and the lockdown policies of various countries have prompted people to have more time to develop deeper relationships with mobile phones and computers. It is obvious that in the post-COVID times, there will be more mobile phones than toilets. They will become an indispensable assistant in people's lives.

Various applications based on smartphones will make smartphones a more important life element in addition to eating, going to the toilet, and sleeping. There will be a greater number of computers, and their functions will be stronger than the human brain. In post- COVID times, mobile terminals will play the role of everyone's indispensable life secretary.

The Future of Man-machine Mix is Coming

The promotion and popularization of 5G have made mobile IoT scenarios with mMTC and uRLLC come true. With the continuous popularization of the intelligent society, computing chips and connection capabilities continue to be embedded in all devices that can be powered on. Sensors will become ubiquitous and outnumber human eyes. Trillions of sensors will be embedded in every corner of society, forming a new scene of the Internet of Everything.

The essence of the Internet of Everything is in line with the big logic that the information technology industry has continued to expand from the cloud to the terminal in the past 50 years. It is a natural extension of the evolution law from services to PCs and laptops to mobile phones. All things are interconnected, intelligent, and constantly being upgraded. The IoT will also greatly expand the penetration rate of information technology in the whole society and improve the entire society's informatization degree and operation efficiency.

In this background, as a smart key that connects people and things, wearable devices will exert their greatest value, that is, to digitize the vitals of the human body. The man-machine mix will become increasingly popular in the future, and ubiquitous smart wearables will connect people with all things. With the help of smart wearables, the physical functions of the human body, from the external functional limbs of the human body to the internal organs, will be significantly expanded.

For example, with the help of invisible smart wearable glasses or smart eyes, our visual sensory functions are expanded; with the help of robotic limbs, our limb functions are expanded. Normally, the weight of the items we carry in our hands or the weight of heavy objects we can bear is limited. Still, with the help of intelligent wearable robotic limbs, our load-bearing capacity can be considerably stronger. Soon, we will be able to implant chips to track our vitals at all times and keep our health management online all the time. For example, part of the functions of our internal organs will be replaced by smart wearables, such as heart pacemakers, contraception for men and women, tumor monitoring, etc.

In addition, wearables will become a new entrance to the mobile network, leading to the overall upgrade of the personal area network. They are attractive because they can free humans from the constraints of computers and smartphones and enable new mobile web portals.

The mobile network that relies on smartphones is still relatively limited. Smartphones act as network servers and input and output terminals; however, the introduction of wearables will change this situation. In the future, smartphones will only serve as networking servers, while wearables will become the input and output terminal of the mobile network, freeing people's hands and allowing them to access the Internet anytime, anywhere.

For example, by automatically inputting human health and exercise status through smart watches and outputting 3D images with excellent visual effects through smart glasses, people's life, work, and entertainment experience will undergo revolutionary changes. Wearable technology is about to enter the lives of ordinary people on a large scale. It will be at every corner of life, bringing significant technological changes to human beings. But it is foreseeable that the metaverse era will not officially arrive before 2035 because the period before 2035 still has the basic carrier technology in the metaverse, that is, the period of improvement and development of the wearables industry. It is expected that by the middle of this century, with the development of the wearables industry, the physical functions of the human body will be significantly expanded, including the human sexual lifestyle, which will undergo drastic changes in form. Remote virtual sex will take place.

From the Internet to the IoT

From the P.C. Internet to the mobile Internet and to the Internet of Things (IoT), all rounds of the information revolution point to the same keyword—"connection." If the

Internet is considered to have bridged the connection between "people and people" and "people and information," the IoT goes one step further and comprehensively connects "people and things" and "things and things." Certainly, the development of the IoT has also experienced a long period of introduction, accumulation, and verification.

In 2008, the first International Internet of Things Conference was held, where the number of IoT devices exceeded the number of attendants for the first time. The introductory stage of the IoT was characterized by the introduction of related concepts of the IoT and the connection of early IoT devices. In 2013, Google Glass was released, revolutionizing IoT and wearable device technology. In 2016, various elements that would shape the ecosystem of the IoT industry were ready. The initial period of the IoT mainly involved trial and error and resulted in some sensing and communication technologies.

As soon as the various elements of the IoT industry chain were basically in place, the scale effect of the IoT on the transformation of the national economy and industry could be seen. 2018 to 2019 was the opening period for the market to verify the implementation of IoT technology solutions. During the IoT verification period, the drive from technology, policies, and industry giants still played a significant role in the development of the IoT industry. However, it could not be ignored that the influence of market demand factors was expanding.

Since Kevin Ashton proposed the term "Internet of Things" in 1999, it has gradually evolved from an embryonic form to a new engine that drives global economic growth. The new wave of technology has knocked open the door to a new age and set a unique tone for it.

Although from the perspective of the connected objects, the IoT merely adds a variety of "things," it has an extremely far-reaching impact on the expansion and sublimation of the connotation of the connection. The IoT is no longer a single connection center of "people." Things can be connected independently without human manipulation, ensuring the objectivity, real-timeness, and comprehensiveness of the content to be delivered via the connection to a certain extent. In addition, the IoT connects every detail of the real world to the network, creating a system where virtuality (information, data, and process) and reality (human, machine, and commodity) reflect and connect one another. The physical entities establish their own digital twin in the virtual world, making the state of itself traceable, analyzable, and predictable.

In the environment of the IoT, on the one hand, everything is an entrance. Besides the data generated from the users' active interaction, many passive user data will be recorded in real-time and without being noticed. Therefore, enterprises can understand user needs comprehensively, three-dimensionally, and dynamically. On the other hand, intelligent factories in the age of the IoT can quickly meet users' continuously iterative needs for customization through flexible production lines and transparent supply chains.

Compared with the approximately five billion devices accessing the mobile Internet, the scale of IoT connections will be at least an order of magnitude bigger, covering everything from wearable devices, smart homes, autopilot vehicles, connected factories, and smart cities. In the future IoT age, the devices connected to the network will be more intelligent and data applications richer without being limited to their current simple item status and location information. This new wave that the IoT leads will fundamentally change the way of life we are used to and reshape the pattern of the global industrial economy.

The IoT Extends the Internet

The Internet is the foundation of the IoT, while the IoT is an extension of the Internet. The proposal and application of the IoT make it possible to communicate between people and things and between things effectively. Ultimately, it is expected to realize the vision of a highly intelligent IoT ecosystem. Therefore, though the IoT, as a young concept, has only developed for about 30 years, the whole world attaches great importance to it.

As the integration and comprehensive application of a new generation of information technology, the IoT will trigger a new round of industrial transformation. It is a new driver for economic growth. As computer technology and communication technology mature, many countries and regions such as Japan, the U.S., South Korea, and the E.U. have put forward the development strategy of the IoT as the main driving force for future economic development.

To grasp the initiative of future economic and technological advancement, China has made a strategic layout in the field of IoT and has continued to widen its policy support for it. In May 2011, the Ministry of Industry and Information Technology issued the first *China IoT White Paper*, which comprehensively analyzed the opportunities and challenges faced by China's IoT; it was pointed out in *The Twelfth Five-Year Plan* and *The Thirteenth Five-Year Plan* that China shall make remarkable achievements in the core technology of IoT and its industrial application, implement the strategy of making the country stronger through the Internet, accelerate the construction of a digital China, and promote the comprehensive integration and penetration of the IoT into various industries.

According to the *2020 China IoT White Paper* of the China Academy of Information and Communications Technology, the number of IoT connections in China accounts for 30% of the world's total. In 2019, the number of IoT connections in China was 3.63 billion, of which the number of mobile IoT connections accounted for a large proportion, which had increased from 671 million in 2018 to 1.03 billion by the end of 2019. By 2025, the number of IoT connections in China is expected to reach 8.01 billion, with a compound annual growth rate of 14.1%.

The IoT can be divided into the perception, network, and application layers per the technical framework.

The perception layer, as the bottom layer of the IoT, is considered to be the foundation of the application and development of the IoT. It is responsible for information acquisition and is composed of basic chips, sensors, and radio frequency components. The network layer efficiently transmits the information obtained by the perception layer through communication technology and is considered the core of the Internet of Everything. Its key technology is communication between things, including wired and wireless transmission.

The application layer applies IoT technology to all walks of life. Obviously, with IoT being a new generation of information technology, the terminal application scenarios of the IoT industry are so broad that all aspects of social production and life are involved.

Furthermore, the application layer is roughly divided into three main threads; the consumer IoT oriented at the demand side, the productive IoT oriented at the supply side, and the smart city application IoT. According to GSMA Intelligence (the definitive source of mobile industry insights, forecasts and research, used around the world), from 2017 to 2025, the number of connections in the Industrial IoT (both productive and smart city) will increase by 4.7 times and that of consumer IoT by 2.5 times.

In fact, for a long time in the past, IoT applications have been lightweight. But, with the promotion of 5G, the heavyweight IoT will be applied, such as the interconnection of thousands of screens or edge computing.

Edge computing is an essential difference between 5G and 3G/4G. It migrates the cloud computing platform from the core network element to the edge of the wireless access network close to the terminal. It supports the mobile access network to build a processing platform close to users and terminals. The platform provides I.T. or cloud capabilities to reduce the multi-layer delivery of services and the burden on the core network and transmission.

In short, the edge computing architecture allows data to be exchanged only between the source data device and the edge device instead of uploading all of it to the cloud computing platform. It gives data devices the right to generate and transmit large amounts of data. Obviously, in the future IoT era, the devices connected to the network will be more intelligent and data applications more abundant, instead of being only limited to the current simple item status and location information.

Nowadays, the development momentum of the IoT continues to be enriched, the industry generally recognizes the market potential, the development speed is accelerating, technological and application innovations keep emerging one after another, and the rapid development of the IoT has become inevitable. As the IoT is explicitly positioned as an essential part of China's new critical infrastructure that supports the development of the digital economy, while the IoT is building an intelligent connection of everything, we can embrace a world like never before.

Therefore, it is expected that by 2035, the market demand and usage of sensors for monitoring purposes will be at least three times greater than today. This is going to be an industry with enormous commercial value. China's investment in urban (environment and people) surveillance and monitoring will be more than double that of Western countries in the same period, and their popularization rate will be much faster than that in Western countries. Under the restriction of citizens' privacy rights, western countries will have a slower process of digital city construction to a certain extent. Still, the trend of IoT for commodities is unstoppable.

4.2 The Digital Twin Bears Human Ambitions

Technology is not only a label of an era but the industrial changes it leads to making this era.

In the digital age, the digital twin, as one of the most critical digital technologies, is irreplaceable in the digitization of the human society and therefore is frequently discussed in the keynote speeches at major summits and forums, attracting great attention both inside and outside the industry.

Earlier in New York, Microsoft C.E.O. Satya Nadella called the digital twin one of the biggest tech trends. Gartner, a world-renowned I.T. research organization, listed digital twin as one of the top ten emerging technologies for three years in a row from 2017 to 2019.

With the maturity of the idea of the digital twin and the advancement of technologies, a world of digital twins is under construction, from components to complete machines, from products to production lines, from production to services, and from static to dynamic. Based on the maturity of sensors, intelligent equipment, industrial software, the industrial Internet, the IoT, cloud computing and edge computing, and the accumulation of broader business practices, the digital twin has reached a new time node.

The digital twin transfers the real data to the virtual space in real-time, thus providing a virtual base for the realization of the digital, intelligent, and networked industrial model. Also, they bear the ambition of human beings and draw a clearer and clearer path to explore their future imagination.

Conceptual Evolution of the Digital Twin

The concept of the digital twin was born in the U.S. In 2002, Michael Greaves, a professor at the University of Michigan, proposed the concept of virtual digital expression equivalent to physical products in the course of product life cycle management: a digital replica of a specific device or a group of devices that can abstractly express the real one/ ones and be used as a basis for testing under actual or simulated conditions. The concept stems from the desire to express more explicitly the information and data of the devices, hoping to gather all the information for more advanced analysis.

NASA's Apollo project, from many years before, truly put the digital twin concept into practice. NASA needed to build two identical space vehicles, with one staying on Earth as the twin. It was used to reflect (or mirror) the state of the spacecraft performing a mission.

Today, many mainstream companies in the industry have given their understandings and definitions of the digital twin, but people's understanding of it keeps evolving.

The evolving understanding is seen in Gartner's discussion of the digital twin in the past three years. In 2017, he defined a digital twin as a dynamic software model of an object or system through which billions of physical objects will be expressed within three to five years. In the emerging technology maturity curve, in 2017, Gartner released the digital twin was in the nascent stage of innovation and five to ten years away from mature applications.

In 2018, he defined it as a digital expression of a real-world object or system. With the wide application of IoT, digital twins can connect real-world objects, provide information on their status, respond to changes, improve operations, and increase value.

In 2019, his definition of a digital twin changed into a digital mirror image of an object, process, or system in real life. Large systems such as power plants or cities can also create their digital twins.

In the process of maturation and improvement of the digital twin concept, its main applied agents are no longer limited to the insight and improvement of product performance based on the IoT but extend to broader fields, such as digital twins of factories, cities, and even organizations.

Horizontally, on the model dimension, from the perspective of model requirements and functions, some people believe that a digital twin is a three-dimensional model, a copy of physical entities, or virtual prototypes. On the data dimension, some believe that data is the core driving force of a digital twin with a focus on its value in product life cycle data management, data analysis and mining, data integration, and fusion, etc.

On the connection dimension, some believe that a digital twin is an IoT platform or industrial internet platform. This view focuses on perceptual access from the physical world to the virtual world, reliable transmission, and intelligent services. For services, there is one voice that digital twin is a simulation, virtual verification, or visualization.

There are many different understandings of a digital twin without a unified definition. Still, physical entities, virtual models, data, connections, and services are the core elements of a digital twin.

Broadly, a digital twin creates a digital virtual model based on the physical entity of a device or system. This virtual model will render services on the information platform. It is worth mentioning that, unlike computer-assisted drawings, the most significant feature of the digital twin is its dynamic simulation of the physical object. In other words, it "moves."

Meanwhile, the basis for the "movement" of the digital twin is the physical design model of the physical object, the "data" fed back by the sensors, and the data of historical operation. The real-time state of the object and the external environmental conditions will be "connected" to the "twin."

From Virtual Reality Mapping to Full Life Cycle Management

It is based on the core elements of the digital twin and the matching social needs that make the digital twin, as a concept beyond reality, a digital mapping system of one or more essential and interdependent equipment systems. The popularity of the digital twin is rising in post-COVID times.

The real-virtual mapping is the fundamental feature of the digital twin. It realizes bidirectional mapping between the physical and digital twin models by constructing a digital twin model for the physical entity. This plays a vital role in improving the performance and operation of the corresponding physical entities.

In fact, for future intelligent fields such as the industrial Internet, smart manufacturing, smart cities, and smart medical care, virtual simulation is a necessary link. The primary characteristics of real-virtual mapping of a digital twin pave the path for industrial manufacturing, urban management, medical innovation, and so on to transform from "heavy" to "light."

Taking the Industrial Internet as an example, in the real world, to repair an enormous piece of equipment, it is necessary to consider matters like the profit and loss of a shutdown, the complex structure of the equipment, and arranging personnel to conduct on-site inspections. It is an obviously "heavy project." With the digital twin, repairmen only need to feedback data to the digital twin to judge the condition of the actual physical equipment and complete the inspection and repair.

With the concept of a digital twin, General Electric proposed one way to integrate physical machinery and analysis technology and applied it to the manufacturing of its aero engines, turbines, and M.R.I. equipment, so that every piece of equipment has a digital twin, thus realizing accurate monitoring, fault diagnosis, performance prediction, and control optimization of the operation and maintenance processes.

During the COVID-19 pandemic, the world-famous Leishenshan Hospital was built using a digital twin. The Central-South Architectural Design Institute (C.S.A.D.I.) was ordered to design the second Xiaotangshan Hospital in the Wuhan—Leishenshan Hospital, in Wuhan, Hebei province in China. The building information modeling (BIM) team of C.S.A.D.I. created a digital twin for Leishenshan Hospital via BIM.

According to the project requirements, BIM was used to guide and verify the design, which was strong support for the design and construction.

The construction of digital twin cities in recent years has ignited transformative innovations in intelligent urban management and services. For example, the Xiong'an New Area in Hebei Province, China (about 100 km southwest of Beijing) has an amazing digital twin of an urban underground integrated pipe system that integrates 12 types of municipal pipelines, including underground water supply pipes, renewable water pipes, hot water pipes, and electric power communication cables; the digital twin city of

Yingtan in Jiangxi Province won the Global Smart City Digital Transformation Award at the Barcelona Global Smart City Conference.

In addition, since the real-virtual mapping is a dynamic simulation of physical objects, it means that the digital twin model continues to grow and enrich itself: throughout the product life cycle, from product demand information, helpful information, material information, service environmental information, structure information, assembly information, process information, test information to maintenance information, it continues to expand, enrich, and improve itself.

The more complete the digital twin model is, the more it can approximate its corresponding entity to visualize, analyze, and optimize the entity. When the various digital twin models of the product life cycle are compared to scattered pearls, the chain connecting these pearls is the digital thread. The digital thread can connect not only the digital twin models of various stages but the complete product life cycle information, thus ensuring the consistency of various product information when changes occur.

In the full life cycle field, Siemens has extended the value of the digital twin to many industries with the help of the Product Lifecycle Management (P.L.M.) and has achieved remarkable results in medicine and automobile manufacturing.

Taking GlaxoSmithKline's vaccine R&D and production laboratory as an example, the complex vaccine R&D and production have finally achieved a total virtual whole-process twin monitoring through the complete construction of a digital twin. The company's quality control expenditure decreased by 13%, with 25% less rework and scrap, saving 70% on compliance costs.

From real-virtual mapping to full lifecycle management, the digital twin covers various application scenarios for various industries. In 2018, the article *Digital Twins and Their Application Exploration on Computer Integrated Manufacturing Systems* (from CNKI. net) summarized the application of digital twins in 11 fields with 45 sub-categories, including aerospace, electric power, automobiles, oil and gas, health care, shipping, urban management, smart agriculture, building construction, safety and first aid, and environmental protection.

This made digital twins a hot cake in digital transformation. The industry white paper *How to Use Digital Twins to Help Enterprises Create Value*, co-published by Gartner and iRootech, predicted that by 2021, half of the large industrial enterprises would have adopted digital twins, increasing their efficiency by 10%, and by 2024, over 25% of new digital twins would have been adopted as binding-ready for new IoT-native business applications.

Towards the Digital Twin Era

The history of industrial development is the history of physical manufacturing. In the past, Edison's trial-and-error method created physical products according to the design blueprint and production process, and experiments and tests were repeated to meet the functional and performance requirements of the products. However, the advent of computers and software has changed it all.

In 1980, Francis Bernard, father of CATIA, a 3D interactive design software of Dassault Systèmes, pioneered the simple solid design of curve design. By operating a light pen, the pattern of manifestation of a 3D surface and the simple entity on the computer screen was far better than in the past, thus laying the foundation for the transformation of the world's industrial design from 2D modeling to 3D modeling.

Subsequently, Dassault Aircraft adopted simple 3D modeling technology to produce aircraft components. From 1986 to 1990, Boeing used it for aircraft assembly verification and set up a significant number of preliminary specifications to guide the use of 3D design. With the enhancement of computer performance, the miniaturization of integrated circuits, and the improvement of computing speeds, the emergence of UNIX workstations considerably lowered the cost of 3D design.

Digital design has evolved from early 2D design to 3D modeling, from 3D wireframe modeling to 3D solid modeling and feature modeling, giving birth to technologies such as direct modeling, synchronous modeling, hybrid modeling, and BIM, oriented in the construction industry.

With the development and application of digital technology, when people apply digital twins to rebuild an object, a system, a city, and even a world, they fully expose human ambitions.

In retrospect of the process of the manufacturing industry digitalization in the past 20-30 years, the digital twin has evolved from the high-end and complex manufacturing industry such as aircraft, automobiles, and ships in the past and the industrial equipment industry that manufactures these products to the high-tech electronics industry, and daily consumption industry, such as clothing, cosmetics, furniture, food, and beverage. There are also more digital twin applications in the infrastructure industry, including railways, highways, nuclear power plants, hydropower plants, thermal power plants, urban construction, and even the entire cities.

At the beginning of 2022, Dassault Systèmes proposed that the digital revolution should expand from the lifeless "thing" in the material world to the living "life." From the creation perspective, the human body is far more complex than machines. The human body has 37 trillion cells, each involving 42 million proteins in its life cycle. Human body digitization is a systematic study based on multi-discipline and multi-profession knowledge related to the human body. It inputs all such knowledge into the digital twin of the human body. This is conducive to reducing the risk of various surgeries, improving their success rate, accelerating drug development, and enhancing the efficacy of drugs.

As a technology, the digital twin has finally expanded from atomic and device applications to cells, hearts, and human bodies. Even in the entire earth and universe in the future, a digital twin world can be reconstructed in virtual cyberspace. Obviously, the growth of the digital twin has undergone the evolutionary process of digitization, interaction, early awareness, early perception, and shared intelligence. Whether it is from aerospace to human health management, from earth governance to country governance or enterprise governance to group governance, from building construction to post-operation management, the digital twin will become the mainstream technology for global governance in the post-COVID times and will lead mankind into the era of digital twins.

It is foreseeable that the global digital twin market scale will have exceeded US\$ 100 billion by 2035, mainly in the government's urban governance, aerospace, military technology, and dynamic management applications of enterprises. The medical application of digital twins will begin to be valued and breed an independent market of over US\$ 100 billion. Still, the security requirements of data management will be further expanded, too.

4.3 Brain-computer Interface Comes True

By inserting a cable in the back of the head, people can roam freely in the computer world and change "reality" by simply thinking about it. Learning knowledge no longer needs to be done through books, videos, and so on and does not take a lot of time, but knowledge is transmitted directly to the brain. The above is what the 1999 classic sci-fi movie *The Matrix* envisioned for us. It seems to be an unrealistic fantasy, but it is a reasonable assumption based on the long-established brain-computer interface technology. And science and technology can make that happen.

In fact, brain-computer interface technology is nothing new. The great scientist Stephen Hawking used it. As brain science, brain nerve study, and computer technology continue to deepen, brain-computer interface technology will continue to mature. It will not only be used by the disabled but will become a standard technology for the human brain read-and-write in the future.

Brain-computer Interface Goes on Stage

It should be noted that the brain-computer interface is essentially a brand-new informa-tion communication and interaction interface. To understand the nature of information communication, it is necessary to understand the language of humans.

Language is the product of higher cognitive activity in the human brain. As N.Y.U. Psychology and Neuroscience Professor David Poeppel wrote in his paper on *Science Advances*, a sub-issue of *Science*, language is how sound waves put information in people's heads.

When people listen to others talk, the ear converts the sound waves into neural signals, which are processed and translated by different encephalic regions. The auditory cortex is the first to be processed. Years of neurophysiological studies have shown that brain waves in the auditory cortex, according to the frequency of changes in the intensity of sound waves, segment and lock acoustic signals. Basically, the brain waves fluctuate in the sound waves like a surfer. The brain is likely to distinguish syllables and identify semantics through changes in the sound waves' intensity to load long language information into sections and convert them into easy-to-process small sections of information.

However, human language did not evolve overnight but over a long period. From neuropeptides, neurons to neural nets; from the ganglion to the fusion of several ganglia to form the brain, and then to the formation of the primitive brain; from the emergence of the reptilian brain that controls body organs and has exquisite division, to the emergence of the limbic system that controls complex emotions such as love, anger, and fear, and then to the emergence of the cerebral neocortex for rational thinking, the nervous system has undergone a development process from 0 to 1, from simple to complex, from low-level to high-level.

It is precisely because the cerebral neocortex of the human brain is good at thinking, especially at abstraction, and can summarize and deduct the essential properties of things that about 100,000 years ago, humans acquired the groundbreaking tool of being able to refer to something concrete with a specific abstract sound.

For example, the pronunciation of the word "stone" is not the stone itself but a representative symbol of the object. And just like that, a protolanguage was born. Soon, all kinds of things in the world had corresponding names. By 50,000 BC, humans were able to communicate using complex language entirely. From then on, language could not only convert all kinds of wonderful ideas in the human brain into a series of sound symbols but transmit them to other people's brains through air vibrations and make them understood.

The emergence of human language has not only marked everything in the world with symbols but also generated an essential function, enabling people to learn things they have not personally experienced and thus gain indirect experience. As a result, the survivability of the human race has been dramatically improved.

It is precisely because of language learning that experience and wisdom have been passed down from generation to generation and accumulated in the tribes' knowledge base, so that future generations can continue to explore the wisdom of their ancestors. In this way, language endows the tribes with a powerful collective intelligence, from which everyone benefits. With the continuous accumulation of knowledge, the continuous improvement of productivity, and the gradual improvement of labor productivity, human beings entered the urban age.

With the evolution of human civilization, great knowledge reserves have created conditions for the human industrial revolution, and technology has also been continuously updated in history. Today, people have entered an era in which information technology develops rapidly, and the continuous breakthrough of A.I. technology makes human beings find themselves inferior to A.I. in terms of learning ability because they cannot acquire knowledge from massive amounts of knowledge quickly.

And this defect arises from languages that have made outstanding contributions to human civilization because human languages are inherently defective in low precision and low efficiency.

From the perspective of language precision, the precision is relatively low no matter what kind of human language. The sociality and ambiguity of language make the communication accuracy between people low so that people have to spend a lot of time on communication. During human-to-human communication, a lot of information is lost. From the perspective of language efficiency, people cannot input objective information into the brain as fast as a computer. When it is transmitted by language and texts, the speed is indeed slow.

And when people entered a new digital age, human weaknesses and limitations began to be magnified. As the wheels of time roll forward, the inherent needs of historical development drive the advancement and development of technology, and at last, the brain-computer interface goes on stage.

The History of the Brain-computer Interface

As a communication control system that does not depend on the normal efferent (carry messages from the brain to an effector organ) pathways of peripheral nerves and muscles, the brain-computer interface can collect and analyze brain bioelectrical signals and build a direct communication and control path between electronic devices like computers and the brain. Though it has only become a hot technology in cutting-edge scientific research in recent years, we find that the overall history of brain-computer interface research is long and complex.

Primarily, the first stage of the brain-computer interface is the theoretical understanding of the brain structure. German neuroscientist Hans Berger first recorded the electrical activity of the human brain in 1924, and in 1927 he published his seminal work on the electroencephalogram (E.E.G.) of the human brain. As the first commonly used method of brain-computer interface technology, E.E.G. neurofeedback has been in use for decades.

Simply put, when the cranial nerves begin to process information, corresponding electromagnetic signals are generated. The electromagnetic model changes reflect the cortical area's current activity. These signals are amplified and coded into signals with information. This allows researchers to analyze the data and use algorithms to infer what the brain intends to express. For these E.E.G.s, people first analyzed their waveforms in the time domain (spike analysis method). Researchers then used a Fourier transform or a wavelet transform to analyze the energy distribution of the E.E.G. signal in the frequency domain (energy spectrum analysis method, which divides brain waves into alpha, beta, gamma, and delta waves).

Since the mid and late 20th century, chaotic dynamics have risen. It has been discovered that due to the natural complexity of cranial nerves, brain waves are more unstable and nonlinear. Therefore, more and more researchers have begun to use the research methods of chaotic dynamics to analyze brainwaves and cerebral cortex structures. And the fractal dimension is one of the chaotic dynamics tools used in brainwave analysis.

The second stage of E.E.G. is the decoding application of brain signals. In 1970, the Defense Advanced Research Projects Agency launched a program to explore brain communication using E.E.G. In 1976, Jacques J. Vidal of U.C.L.A. published groundbreaking theories and technical suggestions on "direct brain-computer communication." He created the standard definition of a brain-computer interface that is still in use today and focused brain-computer interface R&D on neural repair to assist patients in restoring impaired vision, hearing, and movement.

As technology advanced, the first batch of neuro-prosthetic devices for humans appeared in the mid-1990s. Another important milestone year for brain-computer interface research was 1998, when researcher Philip Kennedy first implanted a brain-computer interface device into the human body and obtained high-quality data using wireless dual electrodes. Therefore, the brain-computer interface has attracted more attention, and the fact that it can realize the communication between the brain and the computer without the participation of peripheral nerves and muscles highlights the value of applying this technology to the adjuvant treatment of stroke, epilepsy, and other disabilities.

The third stage of the brain-computer interface is moving from the laboratory to the market. In 2006, a Brown University research team completed the first implantation of a brain-computer interface device in the brain's motor cortex, which was used to control a mouse. In 2012, brain-computer interface equipment performed more complex and extensive operations, enabling paralyzed patients to control the robotic arm to drink, eat, type, and communicate with others.

In the opening ceremony of the World Cup in Brazil in 2014, Juliano Pinto, a high-level paraplegic young lad, kicked off the game with the help of a brain-computer interface and artificial exoskeleton technology; in 2016, Nathan Copeland mind-controlled the robotic arm and shook hands with then U.S. President Barack Obama. In 2017, the BrainGate team realized the control of an implantable functional electrical stimulation device through an implantable brain-computer interface. It used an external computer to repair the connection at the fracture of the original neural circuit so that patients with spinal cord injury can control their arms through brain activity and perform some daily activities themselves.

So far, this closed-loop brain-computer interface manipulation has been essentially approaching the futuristic image that people see in sci-fi films in the past so that the idea of the brain-computer interface as an extension of human organs becoming part of the natural human body is coming true.

The Future of Brain-computer Interfaces

Certainly, the brain-computer interface does not mature overnight.

The rudimentary brain-computer interface is a system that uses signals from cranial nerves to control external devices to meet particular needs. An earlier project funded by the U.S. Department of Defense required a brain-controlled robotic arm, hoping to use a brain-computer method to help wounded soldiers who lost a limb in a war. With the help of brain-computer interfaces and robotic arms, they could take care of themselves.

In mid-2019, Elon Musk announced the first generation of brain-computer interfaces, simply described as a "back of the brain intubation" technology. Through a neurosurgical robot, it can safely and painlessly perforate the skull like minimally invasive ophthalmic surgery, quickly implant a chip into the brain, directly read brain signals through the USB-C interface, and be controlled with an iPhone.

One year later, Musk presented the latest achievement on brain-computer interfaces at a conference, including a simplified coin-sized Neuralink implant and a surgical robot to implant it. The new device from Neuralink is named the Link v 0.9. Compared with the original device, its implantation steps differ little, but its brain-computer interface is smaller and performs better. Like the Apple Watch, its battery can last all day and be wirelessly charged while people sleep.

It is worth mentioning that wireless technology has been applied to implantable medical devices for over ten years. Both pacemakers and deep brain stimulation devices have wireless transmission. Although their bandwidth is not great, data transmission is not massive, and wireless charging is impossible. However, Neuralink's wireless transmission transmits both power and data, which means that as an electronic device, Neuralink is complete, which is progress in electronic design.

The chip Musk showed this time has 1,024 channels, while there were 3,072 channels in its previous version. The 1,024 channels can be understood as 1,024 neural signal collection points. Though fewer channels exist within a given encephalic region and range ($2*1$ cm range of motor cortex), the valuable data collected is not necessarily affected. In addition, the new brain-computer interface paired with a new version of surgical robot looks is a significant improvement compared to the giant machine from the previous year.

It scans the brain's structure, and carefully avoids dangerous regions, so the implantation process does not cause damage to the brain.

Musk also stated at the press conference that in the future, everyone would be able to implant a chip in the brain to solve a series of problems, including memory loss, hearing loss, blindness, paralysis, depression, insomnia, extreme pain, anxiety, addiction, stroke, brain damage, etc.

And this is only the first step. Musk's long-term goal is superhuman cognition, which stems from his concerns about A.I. He believes that humans need to be integrated with A.I. to avoid the worst situation in which A.I. becomes too powerful and destroys humans in the future.

This involves a more advanced brain-computer interface that can transform one's own consciousness and memory under human control and conduct two-way communication with the external world (the Internet or personal server). And the human brain can also become a node server with limited access for information transfer.

A more advanced brain-computer interface is an enhancement for humans. Through it, we can gain a lot of knowledge and skills quickly, thus having a superpower unattainable to ordinary humans.

Memory transplantation is the focus of research in this field. At present, American scientists, having discovered the memory code of the hippocampus of the brain, have begun to use the chip to back up the memory and implant the chip into another brain to transplant memory. This experiment was a success in monkeys. Ultimately, this technology aims to transmit a great deal of information and data to the brain through a brain-computer interface, or upload the brain's consciousness to the computer, and immortalize human consciousness and memory in the computer world.

When the brain-computer interface dives to a deep level, it truly combines human and machine as Musk envisions; that is, humans can communicate with each other without language. E.E.G. signals in the brain alone suffice to bridge the communication and realize "lossless" brain information transmission. The essence of this brain-brain interaction is the activity of neuron groups. Unlike the ambiguity of language and the failure to convey a message through words, it is a thorough, undistorted understanding.

In fact, the brain-computer interface, as an emerging technology, has already stood at the forefront of the times. Meanwhile, in addition to technical barriers, it faces the inevitable torture of traditional ethics. In the future, people will apply brain-computer interface to directly input the knowledge that people need to memorize, such as the vocabulary for IELTS and TOEFL, and pure cramming will become increasingly unimportant. However, as brain consciousness is affected by the reading and writing of a brain-computer interface, ideological education will also become the center of attention in various countries.

By 2035, brain-computer interfaces will have achieved a remarkable breakthrough and relatively rudimentary applications. By the middle of the 21st century, it will no longer be limited to the current level of brain consciousness controlling the body or manipulating brain consciousness. Still, it will gradually link with computers and the Internet. With the help of brain-computer interfaces, we can establish connections with mobile phones, computers, etc., anytime and anywhere to solve problems such as knowledge acquisition, analysis, and calculation. And mobile phones will exist in our lives as information processors.

4.4 Autopilot Becomes Mainstream

Only when technology is closely connected with the destiny of mankind can it demonstrate its revolutionary significance. Before A.I., the development of vehicles had gone through several stages: from human feet, the most primitive, to the domesticated horses and donkeys, and carriages, ox carts, etc. Meanwhile, there were sedan chairs and other animal-powered vehicles. Later, with the advent of the steam engine, automobiles and trains replaced the original means of transportation.

With the development of A.I., the value of the smart travel ecosystem related to automobiles is being redefined. The three elements of travel, "people," "cars," and "roads," are endowed with human-like decisions and behaviors, and drastic changes are taking place in the entire travel ecosystem. Substantial computing power and massive high-value data have become the core forces that constitute a multi-dimensional collaborative travel ecosystem. As the application of A.I. technology in the field of transportation becomes intelligent, electric, and sharing, an intelligent transportation chain centered on autopilot will gradually come into being, thus driving human society to the era of smart transportation.

Autopilot Comes True

In August 1925, the first pilotless automobile in human history made its debut. There was indeed no driver in the driver's seat of the car called American Wonder, whose steering wheel, clutch, and brakes operated on their own.

Behind the car was another car, where engineer Francis P. Houdina sent radio waves to control the vehicle in front. They drove through New York's congested traffic, driving from Broadway to Fifth Avenue. With its rigid understanding of autopilot vehicles, this experiment of a "super-large remote control" is still not widely recognized by the industry today.

In 1939, skyscrapers kept springing up in the American territory. People who gradually regained their confidence after the Great Depression had beautiful hopes for the future. At that year's New York World Expo, there was a long queue in front of the Futurama Hall built by General Motors. Crowds flooded in, hoping to see what the "future" looked like.

Designer Norman Bel Geddes explained further in his 1940 book *Magic Motorways* that humans should be removed from driving, and U.S. highways would be equipped with what resembles train tracks to facilitate autopilot systems for automobiles; once the car goes on the road, it would follow a specific route and program, and return to human driving when off the road. He pictured this to come true in 1960.

The reality was cruel. The difficulty was soon recognized in the 1950s when researchers began experimenting as he had envisioned. But after that, technical explorations to achieve autopilot had started everywhere.

In 1966, intelligent navigation first appeared at the Stanford Research Institute (S.R.I.). Shakey, developed by the Artificial Intelligence Research Center of the S.R.I., is a wheeled robot with built-in sensors and software systems. It created a precedent for automatic navigation.

In 1977, the Tsukuba Engineering Research Laboratory in Japan developed the first self-driving automobile based on cameras to detect markings ahead or navigation information. This means that people have started considering the prospect of autonomous vehicles from a visual perspective. Navigation and vision together buried the idea of ground tracks.

In 1989, Carnegie Mellon University took the lead in using neural networks to guide self-driving automobiles. Even though the server of the refurbished military ambulance driving in Pittsburgh was the size of a refrigerator, and its computing power was only 1/10 that of an Apple Watch, in principle, this technology is more or less the same as today's self-driving automobile control strategy.

Similar to the global development, since the 1980s, China has also started research on smart mobile devices, and its initial project also originated from the military. In 1980, China launched the Remote-controlled Anti-nuclearization Reconnaissance Vehicle project, and the Harbin Institute of Technology, Shenyang Institute of Automation, and National University of Defense Technology participated in the research and manufacture of this project. In the early 1990s, China developed its first actual self-driving automobile.

Since 2000, smart automobile features have started to appear. G.P.S. and sensors provide data and application support and readiness for the emergence of self-driving automobiles. Since the popularization of G.P.S., various technologies and automobile manufacturers have accumulated massive data on personal travel, enabling A.I. to learn driving essentials. Automation sensors would allow automobiles to have local real-time sensing and judgment capabilities. For example, automobiles' Anti-locking Braking System (A.B.S.), airbags, and Electronic Stability Control (E.S.C.) have functionally contributed to improving automobile comfort and safety. And the real automobile intelligence commenced in the second decade of the 21st century. With Google's pioneering efforts in A.I. technology, A.I. applications to cars appeared one after another. Their main functions are in areas such as lane changing, parking, etc.

The Present and Future of Autopilot

In the description of autonomous vehicles, the six levels according to the Society of Automotive Engineers (S.A.E.) are no automation, driver assistance, partial automation, conditional automation, high automation, and full automation.

L0 or **no automation**, is the stage where the driver has absolute control.

L1 is called **driver assistance**. In L1, the system has at most partial control simultaneously, either controlling the steering or the accelerator or braking. When emergencies take place, drivers must be ready to take over immediately. Also, humans need to monitor the surrounding environment.

L2 is **partial automation**, is different from L1. The control transferred to the system in L2 changes from partial to complete. That is to say, in a typical driving environment, the driver can transfer both horizontal and vertical control to the system at the same time. And humans need to monitor the surrounding environment.

L3 is **conditional automation**, means that the system performs most of the driving operations. In this stage, the driver gives an appropriate response as per the situation only when an emergency situation occurs. At this point, the system replaces humans to monitor the surrounding environment.

L4, or **high automation**, refers to the stage where the autopilot system can complete all driving operations without the driver making a response. However, now, the system only supports some driving modes and cannot be adapted to all scenarios.

L5 is **full automation**, whose main difference from L0, L1, L2, L3, and L4 is that the system can support all driving modes. During this stage, the driver may no longer be allowed to be the controlling subject.

From the perspective of technological development, most smart driving technologies in China and abroad are between L2 and L3. It is worth mentioning that with L3, compared with L2, after the autopilot system is activated, the vehicle will completely handle all ride-related problems, including acceleration, deceleration, overtaking, and avoiding obstacles. This also means that in the event of an accident, the responsibility confirmation will change from a person to a vehicle.

L3 is a connection link for autopilot. The autopilot technology of L3 is an essential parting line to distinguish between "pilot" and "autopilot" and the transition between unadvanced driver assistance and advanced driver assistance.

L2 autopilot is centered on human beings, and its autopilot system is only an assistance. L2 mostly corresponds to the current common A.D.A.S. (advanced driver assistance systems), including A.C.C. (adaptive cruise control), A.E.B. (autonomous emergency braking), and L.D.W.S. (lane departure warning system). It still must be the human driver that steers the vehicle.

L3 is the true autopilot. The autopilot system completes most of the driving judgments and actions. The system drives the car under certain conditions, but it is still up to the driver to make decisions when there is an emergency. And the so-called conditions include several functional elements: highway pilot (HWP, 0-130 km/h), traffic jam pilot (TJP, 0-60 km/h), automatic valet parking, high-precision map + high-precision positioning.

The rise of autopiloted vehicles is inseparable from the boom in A.I. The process of a human driving a car is divided into the following steps: first, observe the surroundings and traffic lights, and then accelerate/decelerate, turn/switch lanes through the accelerator, brakes, and steering wheel according to the intended destination direction, and the operation of pulling over. This process is subdivided into perception, decision-making, and control layers in the research of autopilot. Therefore, according to the deduction, combining sensors, machines, and A.I. algorithms will outperform human driving.

However, this seemingly flawless deduction has to face a technical dilemma; although there are a combination of sensors that can perform 360° full coverage scans centered on the vehicle; the mechanism intelligence represented by AlphaGo has proven that machines can do a lot better than humans in speed, accuracy, and other aspects; when the machine makes a decision, it transmits the signal to the steering system, braking system, and transmission system of the vehicle through the wire control system, which ensures the speed and accuracy of the signal. Therefore, its perception, decision-making, and control seem to outdo that of a human. However, as the top A.I. scholar, Professor Li Feifei of Stanford University, emphasized in the conversation with historian Yuval Noah Harari, author of *Sapiens: A Brief History of Humankind* and *Homo Deus: A Brief History of Tomorrow*, the world's existence is not two groups, and real society is far more complicated. In addition to algorithms, there are a lot of players and rules. When autopilot research deepens, the problems of sensors, chips, and data gradually surface.

As a device for detecting external road conditions, the information autopilot sensors collect will be used to make driving decisions, which is an essential guarantee for driving decision-making. Without complete information, it is impossible to support decision-making systems to make correct and safe driving decisions. Though many sensors can outperform the human eye in a single indicator, the difficulty of integration and the accompanying cost dilemma has become the first severe test in the evolution of autopilot.

The problem of multiple sensors leads to the hidden danger of the following problem: the chip's performance. Suppose a more comprehensive understanding of external road condition information is required. In that case, more sensors need to be installed, putting forward a higher requirement for integration. In the case of high-speed driving, the data information is more massive due to changes in road conditions information.

According to Intel's calculations, an autonomous vehicle equipped with a G.P.S., cameras, radar, and lidar (Light Detecting and Radar), will generate about 4 T.B. of sensor data to be processed daily. Such a vast amount of data must be supported by powerful computing equipment, and even top GPU companies like N.V.I.D.I.A. have almost reached the ceiling in terms of the balance between computing power and power consumption. Therefore, more dedicated computing platforms have emerged in recent years, including the AI-specific chip T.P.U. put into application by Google, and the B.P.U. launched by China's top start-up company Horizon. Tesla is also investing heavily in the research of autopilot chips. This will be a huge technical hurdle for an autopilot to overcome in a short time.

In addition to the technical bottlenecks at this stage, the autopilot will continue to face commercial and technical challenges in the subsequent commercial development. From a business logic perspective, autopilot can generate the most significant commercial value in first- and second-tier cities or even in the central districts of cities. However, from the current technical conditions, it cannot enter first- and second-tier cities in one step. More tests are needed for verification to ensure its safety and reliability. In short, current road tests are not yet ready to popularize autonomous vehicles.

Once an autonomous vehicle causes an accident on the road, it will face a crisis of trust among users. Therefore, closed-field testing and open road testing of autonomous vehicles in the city's suburbs (or new districts) have become a transitional solution. At present, to ensure the safety of vehicles on the road, autonomous vehicles must undergo simulation tests and closed field tests, and on this basis, open road tests.

Roads Are Redefined

In the process of urbanization, transportation is the lifeblood of economic and social development. Today, how we travel has changed dramatically from what it used to be. Whether it is the diversity of travel modes or the convenience, comfort, and safety of travel, all have been improved. However, we still face many problems such as road congestion, insufficient parking space, and frequent traffic accidents.

The traffic system is characterized by being time-varying, nonlinear, discontinuous, unmeasurable, and uncontrollable. In the absence of data in the past, people studied urban road traffic in a "utopian" state. However, as technologies advance, such as instant communication, the IoT, and big data, it has gradually become possible to collect complete data and analyze transportation. A revolution in the transportation system has arrived.

The coordinated development of intelligent transportation will become a trend, the autonomous control capability of vehicles will continue to improve, and total autopiloting will eventually become a reality. This will change the relationship between people and vehicles, liberating them from driving and enabling them to consume information in the vehicles.

Vehicles will become an information node in the network and exchange massive data with the outside world, thereby changing the interaction mode between the vehicle, people, and the environment. They sense the surrounding information in real-time and derive more forms of information consumption.

In the future, with the popularity of autopilot, most people will no longer need to buy a car of their own. As an on-demand service, travel can fully share resources such as roads and cars, thereby improving the overall operational efficiency of the society.

The development of these AI-based networked vehicles has profoundly changed people's travel behavior. After the hands are liberated from the steering wheel, the applications of entertainment, information, office work, and media simultaneously liberated open up a giant service content market. These new application scenarios will be able to reshape the entire automotive industry and rewrite existing concepts such as car ownership and mobility.

The roads will be redefined. The future roads will be intelligent and digital. Every square meter will be coded, using active radio frequency identification (RFID) and passive RFID to transmit signals. The intelligent traffic control center and the vehicles can read the information in these signals. And through RFID, underground roads and parking lots can be accurately located.

According to the developmental trend of science and technology, the future road traffic system will inevitably break the traditional thinking and focus on exerting the human sensing ability. Vehicle intelligence and automation will be the most basic requirements, traffic accidents will hardly cause casualties, and the traffic capacity of the road network will be significantly improved. Certainly, the basis for all these to come true is to ensure that the communication technology is high-speed, stable, and dependable.

By that time, more advanced information, communication, control, sensing, and computing technology will have been integrated and applied to the maximum extent. The relationship between people, vehicles, and roads will be lifted to a new stage. Transportation in the new era will be remarkably characterized by being real-time, accurate, efficient, safe, and energy-saving. The intelligent transportation system will surely ignite a technological revolution. After 2035, the profession of driver will gradually be replaced by total autopilot. By the middle of this century, human society will have had the chance to enter the era of the autopilot. Meanwhile, a more 3D transportation network will appear, and unmanned low-altitude flight will begin to be applied.

4.5 Technology Leads Education Towards the Future

The invention and innovation of tools have propelled the progress of human history. Similarly, the reform and innovation of educational techniques also promote the progress and development of education. With the rise of information technology such as A.I., big data, and VR/AR, it is popular that technology is applied to education.

Educational Technology Is Trending

It is an inevitable and ongoing fact that technology changes education the way the birth and development of computer technology have rapidly and profoundly changed how human beings live. In the fields of commerce, transportation, finance, production, and so on, computers have been transforming the traditional model, and education is no exception.

The integration of science and technology and education is first manifested in the changes in educational models and techniques. A French scholar named Monaco believes that the reform of education has gone through four main stages: the performance stage, which relies on direct transmission between people; the expression stage, which relies on indirect language and texts; the imaging stage, which relies on sound and image recording; and the information technology stage, which relies on equal interactions between people.

In addition, the education techniques are also different at different stages, including the means of obtaining information, disseminating information, and teaching interaction. Obviously, technology is the key force driving educational reforms, whether it is the evolution of education stages or changes in educational techniques.

In the performance stage, the means of obtaining information are relatively simple. It relies entirely on word of mouth, and the typical representatives of its educational form are private schools, which are small in scale and without individualized education.

In the expression and imaging stages, papermaking, printing, and imaging techniques appeared, thus changing the educational model of word of mouth. Teachers are no longer the only source of information, and there is a possibility of relative separation between teaching and learning. At this time, schools of all levels and types have a certain scale. Public schools mainly serve the majority of people. They advocate a large scale, emphasize high efficiency, and focus on knowledge dissemination. And there is a stable central pattern of teachers, teaching materials, and classrooms, which become the "iron triangle" of education.

Modern information technology has broken through the time and space limitations of the co-located centralized education model. Especially with the emergence of new technologies such as the mobile Internet, A.I., big data, supercomputing, and brain science, the transmission of knowledge has become more efficient and equal, and the teaching techniques and modes have undergone profound changes. The empowerment of information technology has enabled education to develop faster than in any period in recent history.

On the one hand, communication technology has solved traditional education's time and space limitations through information interconnection. In particular, the advantages of 5G, such as high speed, low latency, high density, and high mobility, enable education to achieve spatial interconnection, synchronous teaching, remote control, and cloud storage.

In terms of space interconnection, the support of 5G enables direct connections between physical spaces. With 4K/8K Ultra H.D. video technology, connected physical spaces can be pieced together. With the help of (Extended Reality (XR) (Augmented Reality (AR)\MR\Virtual Reality (VR)) technology, this piecing together can be more natural and merged into a greater space.

Since 5G also has a high transmission rate under high device density, synchronous teaching can conduct various teacher-student and student-student interactions as in face-to-face instruction. In addition, the low-latency advantage of 5G allows students to control equipment remotely, use learning tools, and perform remote experiments; cloud storage of large-capacity resources such as videos is as fast as local storage.

As a result, with the empowerment of information technology, teaching and learning are no longer limited by time and space, and students' learning mode is transformed. *Massive Open Online Courses* (MOOC), mixed learning, flipped classrooms, ubiquitous learning, mobile learning, and other online education modes are inevitable. The COVID-19 pandemic has promoted the development of remote education and accelerated the process of technical intervention in education. With the help of Internet technology, more people worldwide will enjoy a balanced education quality, and the borderless university based on the Internet will promote education towards universal benefits. Influential universities will define their own educational standards, and mutual recognition of elective credits online and offline will become common. Meanwhile, education will no longer have strict age divisions. Instead, it will be common to complete education online regardless of age, time, and place.

On the other hand, the application of new technologies represented by A.I. in education is redefining the value of human knowledge and ability and leading the connotation of education to develop towards precise content, autonomous learning, and interactive teaching.

A.I. empowers teachers, changes their roles, and promotes the transformation of teaching modes from knowledge imparting to knowledge construction. For example, an A.I. teaching assistant is a kind of virtual teaching assistance software that can complete daily tasks on behalf of teachers. It can answer students' questions, grade assignments, and evaluate papers, so teachers have more time for personalized guidance and one-on-one interactions with students.

AI-empowered schools will change the form of school operations, expand learning spaces, improve school services, and build a more learner-centered learning environment. A.I.-empowered education governance will change the way of governance, promote scientific decision-making in education and precise resource allocation, and accelerate the formation of a modern public education service system.

Correcting Education in the Age of Science and Technology

Educational technology is trending. Obviously, it is necessary to adopt some modern instruments and technologies to transform education and promote educational efficiency and quality improvement. But in the meantime, education also follows the ethical contradictions that technical application inevitably faces. In fact, from the history of technological development, human beings will always encounter new problems around the generation and application of various new technologies. These problems are often not limited to technical and application levels but are more humanistic and ethical challenges.

Undoubtedly, technology promises a bright future of improved education, boosting educational efficiency and making education more accessible. But it must be ensured that these techniques can guarantee positive learning outcomes and put human dignity before sloppiness, attrition, and arithmetical measures. The truth is that when people enjoy the convenience brought by technology, they often ignore the social conditions behind it. The harm it brings to education will be unprecedented when technology goes astray.

At the end of 2019, a primary school in Zhejiang Province in China stirred up heated discussions on the Internet for imposing a headband that tests distractions on students. The product manager of the headband claimed that it was a product for training concentration and would help children regulate their brains on their own; the student data collected by the product was fed back to the teachers, who then decided whether to inform the parents of their children's performance.

The misused smart campus system has the same effect as this headband. It was misused by schools, which should have changed the form of school operation, expanded the learning space, improved the school service, and built a more learner-centered learning environment, to run a check-in system, a dormitory management system, a roll call system, a campus surrounding control system, and an intelligent panoramic playground system. In particular, worse than the distraction-preventing headband, the smart classroom system began to emerge in 2018.

Furthermore, all educational products emerging in the market, whether a smartphone app that offers answers to homework exercises or online classes by online tutoring institutions, spend more time on product promotion than product development. Also, profit pursuit has triggered great educational anxiety, thus pushing education away from its original intention.

When technology intervenes in education, people have to rethink the old-fashioned topic—what kind of education is good? Behind the technology, an ideal lifestyle is predicted, and there are the most critical questions people want to know—and the ones that people often overlook.

In other words, in education where technology prevails, people have long been regarding learning outcomes as profit margins, calculating dividends in return on investment in technology and infrastructure, and even treating students as industrial resources to assess their ability to acquire job skills. However, people gradually forget the ability to create meaning through reflection and contextual methods comprehensively. Compared with emotional poetry, technology makes people pay more attention to rational precision.

Education bears too much hope in the integrated development of technology and education. Therefore, between input and output, the cycle should be as short as possible and the gap as small as possible. The practical notion of education is the epitome of utilitarianism and pragmatism. People's pursuit of the external goals of education is higher than pursuing its intrinsic value. Technical rationality has helped education achieve the purpose of delivering "educational products" in a short period, thus turning education into a competition.

Therefore, in the era of science and technology education, as education chases "technological innovation" and "traditional change," the students are passively integrated into this chase. They must constantly adjust their learning to adapt to social and educational changes. In this process, the purpose of education no longer focuses on the enrichment of humanity but only on the adaptation to society and the market.

Relying on technology, education has been domesticated. It has become an industrialized production, a standard component. The school system's education imposes strict and rigid rules to pressure and shape students. The educational purpose of the entire society has become to accelerate the adultization and socialization of children with an emphasis on collectiveness and obedience.

Today, the alienation of technology from education must not be ignored. It further raises the question: why does technology always fail to achieve the goals we set for it in the first place?

The Internet once gave us the hope to change our education so that young people worldwide can enjoy better and more equal education. But the goal is far more ideal than the reality. It's not the fault of the technology but us, who use technology to educate.

Excessive focus on the innovation of technology, and the development of a scientific theory, often makes us forget how it is used—the process in which it is used, the method by which it is used, and the social conditions under which it is used. These are far more important than who invented this technology and who created this theory.

Only by focusing on the process and how technology is applied to education, and what kind of educational ecosystem it can be used can the actual effect of technology be brought into play because the technology is no longer critical during its application but the education. Technology is the tool, while education is the goal.

However, in modern society, children's education is often spoon-fed rather than rational. According to the current education mode, even if the students are well-read, they are not necessarily smart and capable. Education follows the market logic of filling students' heads with knowledge and ignores their judgment and moral cultivation. As a result, from ignorant to learned, students simply go through the change from ignorance of illiteracy to ignorance of literacy.

Education is needed from childhood to adulthood. It should let the educated understand how to move forward step by step and adapt to the changes of the times. As John Dewey put it a century ago, the purpose of education is to enable people to continue to be educated. In other words, the purpose of learning and its reward is the ability to continue growing.

Education is life and the reorganization of all experiences. From beginning to end, people are the starting point of education, and educating people is the ultimate goal of education. Human education must not be bound by technology, nor should it be defined by technology. Education is driven by technology but is not technology. Therefore, education should not only actively embrace new technologies and use technological progress as an effective driving force to reform higher education but also always guard the bottom line of the true meaning of education in the balance and integration of technical rationality and value rationality in education. Throughout, people are the starting point of education, and educating people is the ultimate goal of education. This is also what makes a human being.

From the perspective of educational form, it is foreseeable that by the middle of this century, virtual universities, virtual classrooms, and virtual courses will become the standard education modes of all mainstream universities, and the physical space boundaries of campuses will be broken. Anyone can apply to enter an online university, study its online courses, and obtain the same educational resources, credits, and diplomas as on a physical campus. This will intensify the competition in international education and terribly impact education in developing countries, but it can significantly improve the education level of developing countries.

CHAPTER 5

The Accelerated Arrival of the Era of a Broad Concept of Health

MEDICAL SCIENCE SERVES HEALTH. WITH THE SUPPORT OF MODERN MEDICINE, human longevity continues to be prolonged. Modern medicine has opened up a whole new page, rewriting the relationship between humans and diseases, suffering and death, and the definition of health. The development of modern medicine has separated diagnosis and treatment. As a result, sharper medical technology equipment has been developed, diagnostic theory and terminology keep emerging, and unprecedented scientific research is carried out on the "deep layer" of the human body. Here comes the era of a broad concept of health.

In the era of a broad concept of health, the intelligent medical industry is developing explosively. With the support and application of medical technologies such as blockchains, cloud computing, and artificial intelligence, the development of smart medical care is further promoted. With the rapid development, comprehensive integration, and fast popularization of the new generation of information technology, the foundation of intelligent medical care has been laid. During the COVID-19 pandemic, gene therapy has grown significantly. It will profoundly impact and trigger changes in human life and disease treatment and gradually become a key technology for treating human diseases in the post-COVID times.

In the era of a broad concept of health, assisted reproductive technology will be an essential direction of life science. Genetic screening will evolve from simple screening to artificial fertilization, from embryo transplantation to in vitro uterine environment cultivation. In the next era, human fertility will no longer rely on the human body for conception. The transaction of sperm and eggs will breed a new market, and in vitro fertilization will become a new business. Humanity will also face a future of "living with cancer" and consuming more synthetic foods than natural foods.

5.1 Smart Healthcare Faces Remodeling and Rebuilding

The popularization of technological innovation and the growing healthcare consumption have enabled the intelligent healthcare market to grow steadily. The COVID-19 pandemic has accelerated the cultivation of the demand side of intelligent medical care and rapidly raised consumers' awareness of it. Under the catalysis of the COVID-19 pandemic, from the user end, the server end, to the payers, it is noted that every element of the intelligent medical industry has undergone positive and long-term changes. The COVID-19 pandemic has become a catalyst for the growth of intelligent medical care and will reshape and rebuild the global medical system.

Changes in the medical industry

The development of the medical industry concerns the national economy and people's livelihoods. It is closely related to the health of the people. Presently, countries are confronted with industrialization, urbanization, an aging population, constant changes in the disease spectrum, the ecological environment and lifestyle, and the development of medical and health services face new challenges. Meanwhile, information technology represented by Internet technology is on the ascendant. Internet technology has opened up a second space for human life and promoted the transformation of production relations in various fields of society, like the rise of the digital economy and virtual social interaction. Derivative products supported by intelligent technology have gradually penetrated into all walks of life, and intelligent medical care is no exception.

From the user side, the advantages of intelligent medical care are apparent. The COVID-19 pandemic has significantly accelerated the penetration of intelligent medical care into the C-end. Online communication and consultation can avoid face-to-face contact and high-risk groups gathering while effectively sharing the workload of offline hospitals, thus helping to solve many dilemmas in pandemic prevention and meeting the needs of home treatment and medication for chronic and mildly ill patients under traffic control. Consequently, residents' habits of seeking medical help have been changed.

According to the monitoring data of iResearch, a Chinese consulting agency, from the outbreak of the COVID-19 pandemic in November 2019 to the gradual improvement of the pandemic situation in April 2020, the monthly effective use time of medical and health apps and web pages has increased significantly. A representative example is JD Health. The online consultation on the JD platform was about 50,000 times per day before the pandemic, and it soared to 150,000 times per day during the pandemic. Even after the pandemic was basically controlled in China, it still maintained the level of 100,000 times per day. This pandemic has advanced the market education time for online diagnosis and treatment by at least five to ten years and has led to the rapid development of online medical care in the U.S.

The server end has undergone a transition from conservative to proactive. The Chinese central government highly affirms the vital role of intelligent medical care in the fight against the COVID-19 pandemic. It therefore encourages local governments and public hospitals to render smart diagnosis and treatment services. With the encouragement and support of the policy, public hospitals and doctors that used to be more conservative about the Internet are embracing the Internet. According to the *2020 Digital Health-care Insight Report* recently co-released by BCG and Tencent, before the COVID-19 pandemic, about 170 public hospitals in China could provide Internet hospital services.

As of May 2020, the number had exceeded 1,000. Regionally, there are currently ten provinces, including Heilongjiang, Ningxia, Shanxi, and Sichuan operating regionalized Internet hospital platforms.

Meanwhile, the *2020 Digital Medical Insights Report* also shows that under the influence of the COVID-19 pandemic, more than one million doctors (the total number of domestic doctors is over two million) have begun to provide diagnosis and treatment services through third-party platforms or Internet hospitals. For example, Alibaba Health, the leading Internet medical platform in China, released its *2020 Internet Doctor Ecosystem Report*, which shows that as of August 2020, there were more than 60,000 doctors active on Alibaba Health Internet Hospitals, a year-on-year increase of 40%.

During the COVID-19 pandemic, many countries have also launched digital anti-COVID measures: China has increased investment in information and communication technology infrastructure and enabled A.I. health care services to help with diagnosis and data analysis; the National Health Services (N.H.S.) of the U.K. has cooperated with American tech companies, such as Amazon, Microsoft, and Palantir to build effective digital models to optimize the allocation of medical resources such as ventilators, hospital beds, and medical staff. In addition, the increased demand for medical services due to strict social distancing measures and limited resources for outpatient services has made digital health platforms increasingly popular.

Meanwhile, more families are utilizing intelligent medical devices. During the COVID-19 pandemic, the data connected by smart medical devices and the mode of online doctor services have been further verified, and a large amount of medical and health data has been collected and applied. With the development and popularization of 5G, intelligent home medical devices will become a new traffic entrance with the family as the scene. Women, infants, and new chronic patient groups are its main customers, and leading manufacturers are its key partners.

In general, the operational efficiency of intelligent medical care has been dramatically improved, and the industry reshaped. It is expected to usher in further developmental opportunities through the public-private partnership model in the future.

Optimize the allocation of medical resources

Before the era of intelligent medical care, the treatment mode used to be around the hospital, and doctors were only one technical configuration in the hospital. Under the current hospital-focused medical model, patients with both major and minor illnesses must go to the hospital in person and queue up for consultation and tests. It is common that it is difficult for patients to book an appointment and that hospitals are overcrowded, inefficient, and render low-quality medical services, especially in some populous countries.

Obviously, the true medical core should not be the hospital but the doctors. Intelligent medical care will significantly improve this situation. With the help of the Internet, clinics can be virtualized, that is, online consultation and telemedicine that some companies are trying.

Primarily, regarding online consultation, this virtualization most directly solves the time and space limitations of the offline diagnosis mode. Specifically, in the current hospital treatment system, we must go to particular places and wait in a long queue at an exact time to see some specific doctors. However, with the help of online consultation, patients can consult relevant professional doctors anytime and anywhere, have themselves tested as required for further diagnosis in any qualified hospital, and transmit these reports to the online consultation system. In the meantime, patients can also describe their medical conditions in detail. After receiving the test report and condition description of the patients, doctors make the diagnosis at any time and send the diagnosis results and prescription to the patients.

Indeed, for some special patients, doctors can also conduct online video diagnoses as agreed and give the diagnosis results and corresponding treatment plans. Next, the patients can buy the prescribed medicines at any local pharmacy, clinic, or hospital, and the doctors in the local community clinic assist in using the medicine.

However, in this process, how much doctors should charge for the consultation fee is an unavoidable problem. This determines whether they are willing to spend their personal time serving the patients of the entire country. Therefore, online consultation also needs to establish a set of clearly marked diagnostic costs. Even if it is consultation, different doctors, problems, and needs should have corresponding charging standards, such as which are free, which are charged, and how much is charged.

As a market-oriented product, online consultation must be adjusted by market-oriented means. Certainly, the platform can manage and evaluate the services of doctors. This will release the current medical resources to a large extent, and the relatively market-oriented income will stimulate the enthusiasm of doctors in online consultations as well as their enthusiasm to improve their medical levels.

In addition, there is also telemedicine, which focuses more on the interaction between medical institutions. For example, suppose a patient in Shanghai cannot grasp the specific condition and treatment plan during the local consultation while there are expert doctors in Hong Kong. At this point, a consultation can be conducted through telemedicine.

Also, remote surgery is part of telemedicine. For example, suppose there is a top cardiologist in the world in Boston, but for various reasons, he cannot come to Shanghai and perform surgery on the patient. At this time, as long as the surgical doctors in Shanghai put on smart medical devices such as Google Glass, the American doctor can watch the entire surgery in real-time and guide the Chinese doctors in the operating room to perform the surgery in real-time. Moreover, with the help of telesurgery robots, the American doctor can operate equipment in the U.S. to achieve remote surgery on a Chinese patient.

Indeed, when medical robots are advanced in the future, surgeries with general characteristics may no longer need to be performed by humans but entirely by robots.

Finally, for both doctors and patients, medical staff must provide help and services to patients once the treatment begins. Whether it is treatment at the hospital, at-home treatment, or in the community, the management of the treatment process and rehabilitation are essential during the treatment. The introduction of intelligent medical care, on the one hand, intelligentizes the internal management system of a specific place like a hospital, and on the other, manages patients throughout the treatment with the help of medical wearables.

This will bring a far-reaching impact and changes to the present hospital management. For example, the inpatient services, management, and needs of major hospitals are difficult to keep up with the patients' needs. At the same time, the introduction of intelligent medical care can separate medical care. Nursing will be conducted by specialized institutions that can connect doctors and patients with the help of wearables, the Internet, big data, cloud platforms, and other technologies and provide medical care according to the needs of both parties.

With the help of intelligent technologies such as the Internet, telemedicine, surgical robots, etc., the global medical resources will go through the same rebuilding and re-division of labor of the global industrial chain in the last century, and all countries in the world will exploit their respective advantages in the medical industry chain. The medical industry is therefore expected to have its own industrial chain.

It is foreseeable that by around 2035, the world will have initially built a diagnosis and treatment industry chain with advantageous resource sharing with the help of Internet technology. This will further narrow the gap between medical treatment and diagnosis in different countries. And this global diagnosis and treatment platform will be constructed by entrepreneurs in the U.S., Europe, or China. Currently, there are corresponding basic applications in the U.S. and China, but it will take some time to improve, expand, and integrate. At the same time, the development of Internet medical care in Europe still needs to be accelerated.

With the help of the global Internet diagnosis and treatment platform, the integration and distribution of advantageous medical resources on a worldwide scale can happen. For example, Germany's surgeries are advanced in the world, so it is possible to employ remote surgical robots to hand over some complex surgeries to German doctors to perform through this Internet medical platform; India has the best advantage in the interpretation of X-ray film, so the patient's X-ray film can be transmitted to India with the help of the Internet system, and Indian doctors will interpret and give conclusions. With the help of the globalization of the Internet medical platform, doctors in various countries will become more professional specialists in the medical industry chain and rely on it to render the best quality medical services for people worldwide.

In the era of disease prevention

In the traditional 3D treatment, due to the constraints of technical means, most patients usually choose to go to the hospital when they clearly have physical discomfort. For example, women with breast cancer do not go to the hospital until it develops to a later stage when they notice some symptoms. And the results of the diagnosis at this time are easy to guess. Probably, the best time for treatment has been missed, and the cost and difficulty of treatment have risen sharply.

With the help of medical wearables, sensors are implanted in women's bras to monitor changes in their breasts. Once there are signs of breast cancer, the sensors can promptly remind them to go to the hospital for diagnosis, conditioning, and treatment. For women, this is highly necessary.

Usually, a person is unaware of symptoms such as angina pectoris or severe arrhythmia. Especially when sleeping deeply at night, we cannot perceive a heart rate, so many deaths caused by heart disease occur during sleep. However, based on the wearables connected with the hospital's backend big data, we can monitor our heart rate anytime and anywhere. When it exhibits abnormality, by referring to scientific medical criteria, the system can automatically identify, assess, and diagnose whether the condition is mild or severe through the wearables and even make a prediction.

When people's vital signs change, precursor characteristics often appear in the medical field, so wearables can monitor these precursor characteristics in the human body and make a diagnosis based on the hospital's extensive data system. When the user is in a deep sleep, if the heart rate shows signs of heart disease, the wearables will automatically wake the user or connect to the hospital for an emergency alarm. Apple Watch has a relatively cutting-edge research and applications in medical health monitoring. By around 2035, smart wearables based on vital signs and health management monitoring will have become the standard configuration of human life. They will be no less important than our mobile phones.

Therefore, an important feature of the future of intelligent medical care is to move the current disease treatment model forward to disease prevention. The focus of the entire medical service will shift from short-term acute disease treatment to chronic disease treatment and preventive health care. Also, professionals in health management will be highly valued by the market. Moreover, through the integration of wearables, big data, cloud platforms, and A.I., it is also possible to analyze, predict, and judge users' health by monitoring their daily behavior and diets, and reminding them to make corresponding adjustments in time, to achieve the purpose of disease prevention.

5.2 Contrarian Growth of Gene Therapy

Gene therapy sounds futuristic, but in fact, its use in the treatment of human diseases dates back to the 1970s. In 1972, *Scienc* published the article *Gene Therapy for Human Genetic Disease?*, which formally proposed and was recognized as a treatment for human genetic diseases. In the following decades, the number of studies on gene therapy has exploded. Though gene therapy has had its good days and bad days, after ample research, it has gradually become a common but essential weapon for mankind to fight diseases.

In 2020, the Alliance for Regenerative Medicine released its first-half 2020 report *Innovation Under the COVID-19 Pandemic*. The report pointed out that the field of regenerative medicine (including gene therapy, cell therapy using genetic engineering, common cell therapy, and tissue engineering) has shown excellent resilience in the face of the challenges of the pandemic. In the first half of 2020, the global financing volume completed in this field reached US$ 10.7 billion, exceeding that of the entire 2019. The contrarian growth of gene therapy under the pandemic has demonstrated the breakthrough and promise of life science and technology and will bring more benefits to mankind.

Why do we need gene therapy?

Human diseases can be roughly divided into three types: the first is genetic diseases. The incidence of most genetic diseases is extremely low, usually between one in a thousand and one in a million. The second type of disease is dominated by environmental factors (hardly any by genetic factors), such as bacterial infections, common colds caused by viruses, or bone fractures. The third type of disease is associated with genetic and environmental factors, such as cancer and high blood pressure.

The second type of disease, caused by environmental factors, such as bacterial or viral infection, can be wholly cured thanks to antiviral drugs, antibiotics, and the human body's robust immune system. Similar to cancer, Alzheimer's disease and other third type of diseases dominated by polygenic and environmental factors or genetic diseases are still difficult to be cured with modern medicine.

For genetic diseases, though small molecule drugs and macromolecule antibody-based drugs have achieved great success, the development of these drugs also faces many dilemmas. For example, small-molecule drugs have trouble with tissue distribution and affinity. In contrast, antibody-based drugs primarily target on the membrane surface and are useless for intracellular targets or even nucleic acid targets on chromosomes. Moreover, long-term input of therapeutic proteins is often required to keep the human body stable, which is complicated in process and difficult in development. For many patients, life-long injections are torture.

Therefore, gene therapy was born as a treatment method that can achieve long-term and tissue-specific expression of therapeutic proteins to treat diseases that cannot be treated via traditional drugs or significantly improve treatment. In fact, this seems to be the only hope for many patients in the face of many congenital diseases.

In 1990, a 4-year-old girl named Ashanti with ADA-SCID disease received gene replacement therapy under the breakthrough of many clinical studies since gene therapy was proposed. ADA-SCID is a severe combined immunodeficiency disorder caused by adenosine deaminase (ADA) deficiency. For Ashanti, the world around her is full of danger. Even sharing a glass of water or breathing with others in the same room can kill her.

Scientists used a viral vector as a delivery method and, through in vitro genetic engineering, inserted the healthy ADA gene into her own cells and reinjected the edited cells into her body. Within six months of treatment, Ashanti's immune T cell levels returned to normal. Over the next two years, her health improved, and she had a childhood that was almost the same as her peers.

This case is considered an essential milestone in the history of gene therapy development. Scientists have completed the proof-of-concept of gene therapy through human trials, verifying the safety and feasibility of gene therapy and encouraging more clinical trials to take place. However, the brief brilliance did not last long. In 1999, the first patient to die from it appeared. After gene therapy, the patient exhibited a fatal immune response.

Subsequent series of early trial results exposed severe side effects of gene therapy, including immune responses against vectors and malignant tumors caused by vector-mediated activation of proto-oncogene insertion. These negative results put gene therapy into a slump.

The failed cases have also made researchers begin to reflect on the risk factors of gene therapy, thus promoting the rapid development of more basic research, including virology, immunology, cell biology, animal model construction, and disease-targeted therapy. As these fields developed rapidly, gene therapy gradually crawled out of the predicament in the early 21st century. With ample research, the current gene therapy has steadily been de-stigmatized and has become an essential weapon for humanity to fight diseases.

Three forms of gene therapy

In a narrow sense, gene therapy refers to a treatment method in which functional genes are delivered to patients to correct or replace the virulent genes. In this treatment method, genes of interest are introduced into target cells, and they are either chromosomally integrated with the host cell and become part of its genetic material or stay outside the chromosome without integrating with it. Both are expressed in cells and can treat diseases.

Broadly, any disease treatment method carried out at the nucleic acid level using the ways and principles of molecular biology can be called gene therapy. Therefore, RNA drugs can also count as gene therapy.

At present, there are three primary forms of gene therapy: the first introduces the correct gene into cells to replace the wrongly mutated gene; the second directly repairs the faulty gene, which is often referred to as gene editing; the third modifies cells in vitro through genetic technology, and introduces the edited cells into the body to function.

The introduction of the correct gene into a cell to replace the wrongly mutated gene is called genetic modification or gene augmentation. A vector is first needed to modify a gene to bring genes into cells. The most common vector is viruses that cannot be reproduced after modification because they can integrate genetic sequences into the host genome.

At present, two types of viral vectors are most commonly used, retroviral vectors and adeno-associated viral vectors. Early (1980s to early 1990s) retroviral vectors primarily used gamma-retroviruses and C-type retroviruses; later, scientists developed lentivirus and spumaviruses vectors. These viruses can infect not only non-dividing cells but also carry larger fragments of genes.

These viruses have been engineered to be milder through genetic modification, such as removing enhancers, thus significantly reducing their genotoxicity. The adeno-associated virus vector is not easy to integrate into the host genome, so it is safer. Under this principle, the use of gene therapy has the characteristics of long-term expression and tissue-specific expression of therapeutic proteins. Therefore, there are two paths to designing drugs:

The first adopts gene therapy as a long-acting drug delivery method. The reverse design of gene sequences is performed based on therapeutic proteins to complete drug design, such as the application in wAMD; the second takes gene therapy as a new treatment method. Targeted at incurable or difficult-to-treat diseases, drugs are designed with genes as the starting point, such as Luxtuma or Zolgensma.

Compared with exogenously introduced genes, directly repairing mutated genes is undoubtedly a safer choice. Gene editing is when scientists cut the gene segment that needs to be modified and use the cell's own DNA repair mechanism to change the original DNA sequence of the cell as required.

Gene editing has developed rapidly in recent years, thanks to the discovery of CRISPR, whose greatest amazement is that this pair of gene-editing scissors can receive human programming instructions and only search, bind and cut specific DNA sequences, including human genome sequences. Because of its high efficiency, convenience, and wide application, CRISPR's breakthrough has accelerated genome editing's development.

It should be noted that though the treatment method of gene editing is the ideal design, it has not yet achieved any technical breakthrough. Its operation is challenging, and there is a tremendous ethical controversy when used in germ cells. There is an infamous case where in 2018, He Jiankui of the Southern University of Science and Technology of China was widely criticized worldwide after genetically editing a pair of babies named Lulu and Nana. Though base editing is currently the favorite of the field, gene editing still has a long way to go.

The introduction of genetically modified cells into the human body is the third form of gene therapy, and it is more widely used on tumors. This technology mainly uses CAR-T or T cell receptor-engineered T cells (TCR-T) in the form of ex vivo gene therapy to kill tumors.

For example, CAR-T, a new type of cellular immunotherapy, uses leukocyte separation technology to extract immune T cells from the blood of patients, integrates T cells with a cell that can recognize tumor cells through in vitro genetic engineering technology, activates the chimeric antibody genes of T cells that can kill the tumor cells, and expands the transformed T cells in vitro and infuse them back into the body of cancer patients, to identify and attack their own tumor cells to cure the cancer.

From rare disease to common disease

It is undeniable that gene therapy is beginning to benefit more and more patients who used to be otherwise untreatable in the field of rare diseases.

For example, congenital amaurosis is a rare genetic disorder that occurs within a year of birth. At birth, the baby's eyes neither follow the dolls hanging and swaying, nor look away from the dazzling light source. Slowly, they fall into permanent blindness. Gene therapy is an effective treatment strategy for this disease. Some genes are transferred by placing a viral vector in a tiny area of the retina. In this disease, blind patients can see again as long as the defective gene is corrected.

As for single-gene genetic diseases, such as SCID, sickle cell anemia, hemophilia, thalassemia, and phenylketonuria, gene therapy is also increasingly involved. The principle of treatment is genetic modification. Due to the existence of single gene mutation, target cells will produce abnormal protein or not produce normal protein. Gene therapy introduces a foreign gene into the target cell through a viral vector to express normal protein as a cure.

But in addition to rare diseases, in fact, compared with traditional drugs, which directly supplement important substances (proteins, inorganic substances, polypeptides, etc.) or regulate protein targets in signaling pathways, the role of gene therapy is more "upstream," as it treats the disease at the nucleic acid level. As per the central dogma, diseases caused by abnormal proteins can theoretically be treated by the action of nucleic acids. Based on this, gene therapy can be applied to various fields. In addition to rare genetic diseases, it can also work on more common disease types.

Recently, scientists from the Institute of Molecular and Clinical Ophthalmology Basel (IOB), together with colleagues from the German Primate Center—Leibniz Institute for Primate Research in Göttingen, Germany, have developed a new approach to gene therapy. They used near-infrared light to activate degenerated photoreceptors to restore vision through gene therapy, and their study results were later published in *Science*.

In addition, the first human clinical trial of an experimental therapy by researchers at Seattle Children's Research Institute has brought engineered T cells for type I diabetes closer to clinical practice. A paper in *Science Translational Medicine* shows how the research team used gene editing to target the FOXP3 gene in human T cells. By activating FOXP3, they equipped the T cells with instructions specifically for Treg.

In the era of small molecule drugs, the emergence of macromolecular antibodies has opened the door to a new world, allowing drugs to reach more targets, treat more diseases, and significantly prolong the human lifespan. The emergence of gene therapy has also opened another door for people. Both gene editing and genetic modification provide new treatment options for rare diseases and more possibilities for prolonging human longevity and improving the survival rate.

The maturity of gene therapy and stem cell therapy will profoundly impact and trigger a change in human life and disease treatment. The continuous breakthrough and maturity of genetic technology and stem cell technology will gradually become the key to curing human diseases in the post-COVID times. Indeed, any cutting-edge technology needs to face the test of ethics. From the nature, effect, and gene editing system, we still need to be cautious and thorough. The development of gene therapy can only be sustainable if safety and efficiency go hand in hand.

As gene technology is decoded and scientists from all over the world invest more in its research, it is foreseeable that around 2035, mRNA cancer vaccines based on gene therapy will have become part of life. After people find potential cancer genes through gene sequencing, they can inject corresponding vaccines to prevent cancer lesions in advance. Cancer-targeted drugs based on gene therapy will become the mainstream clinical cancer treatment. Similarly, around the middle of the 21st century, stem cell therapy will no longer be mysterious but will become an essential form of modern medical treatment. Moreover, it will go from professional hospitals to ordinary people's homes, and the stem cell cultivation machine may become as common and essential as a microwave oven.

5.3 Fertility Becomes a New Business

Reproduction is the survival instinct of all creatures and one of the joys of life as a parent. However, with the development of the industrial society and the urbanization of the human society, this rule is being broken.

On the one hand, declining birth rates and population growth in countries around the world have forced the authorities to take measures to encourage childbirth. For example, China recently announced that every Chinese family could have a third child. And the central Chinese government has promised to optimize its childbearing policy further and implement a policy that a married couple can have three kids and its supportive measures.

On the other hand, more and more families suffer from infertility despite their wish to have a child because of the three-child policy. They are a huge group. On average, one in six married couples face such a dilemma, so China has become the world's largest country with assisted reproductive technology (A.R.T.) treatment. There are more than 200,000 IVF cases every year in China.

Under such circumstances, A.R.T. has increasingly become an essential direction of life sciences, enabling markets related to fertility to rise.

Population growth plummets

Over 200 years ago, English economist Thomas Malthus creatively proposed the idea of the Malthus trap. He believes population grows in geometric progression, while food can only grow in arithmetic progression. In this way, if the population expands to a certain extent, there will be food shortages and conflicts between people and land. Therefore, the additional population must always be eliminated in some way, as the population must not exceed the corresponding level of agricultural development.

However, since the beginning of the Industrial Revolution in the West, human beings have succeeded in breaking out of stagnation, boarded the fast train of growth, and jumped out of the Malthus trap. After about 100 years since the Industrial Revolution, the "two highs and one low" (high birth rate, high mortality rate, and low growth rate) in the western population have been gradually replaced by the trend of "three lows (low birth rate, low mortality rate, and low growth rate).

In addition to Western countries, Southeast Asian countries have also fallen into the predicament of low fertility in recent years. The data of the seventh national census in China, which was released not long ago, has stirred up wide public discussion. According to the National Bureau of Statistics, the number of people born in China in 2020 was 12 million, which was less than the 14.65 million births of 2019 by 2.65 million, setting a new low. It was down by 18%. Population growth has fallen off a cliff.

What is more concerning is that the total fertility rate is also dropping. Internationally, when a woman of childbearing age has an average of 2.1 children in her lifetime, that is, when the total fertility rate is maintained at 2.1, the total population of the next generation is ensured not to decline. If it is below 1.5, we may fall into a low fertility trap. With a real fertility rate of 1.4, the Japanese population has declined for over ten consecutive years.

China's fertility rate is lower than Japan's, suggesting that China will soon have a shrinking population. The Chinese Academy of Social Sciences once calculated that should China's total fertility rate remain at 1.6; there would not be negative population growth until 2027. Still, now, its total fertility rate has dropped to 1.3. The negative population growth in China will be happening soon.

Therefore, countries have successfully launched significant policy initiatives to encourage fertility to cope with the aging population proactively. In China, the Political Bureau of the Central Committee of the Communist Party of China convened a meeting on May 31, where it was pointed out that further optimizing the fertility policy, and implementing the policy that a married couple can have three children and its supporting measures will help improve China's population structure, execute the national strategy to respond to population aging proactively, and maintain China's abundant human resource advantage.

Japan is one of the countries with the most severe aging crisis in the world. To encourage fertility, the Japanese government has made great efforts. For example, it provides both prenatal and postnatal welfare. Pregnant women in Japan can enjoy free pregnancy checks, attend free parenting lectures, etc. If their pregnancy lasts more than 85 days (regardless of miscarriage or stillbirth), they can collect a subsidy of JPY 420,000 (about RMB 22,000 or US$ 3,300).

In France, women can apply for unpaid parental leave for up to three years. In addition, French men are entitled to 14 days of fully paid maternity leave when their wives give birth so that fathers can support their spouses and take care of the newborns. Since July 2021, the number of paid days off for French fathers has doubled to 28 to reduce inconvenience for French parents, especially mothers, in scheduling work and housework and stimulate the public's willingness to bear children.

Almost all countries in the world are trying to restore the birth rate. However, in addition to facing the choice of having children or not, there is the dilemma that some families want to but cannot.

The heartbreak of infertility

For example, the *Report on the Status Quo of Infertility in China* shows that there are more than 40 million infertile Chinese couples of childbearing age, accounting for 12.5% to 15% of the population of the childbearing age. Over 20 years ago, the infertility rate among Chinese of the childbearing age was only 3%. One in between six and eight married couples suffers from infertility.

Gestation is the proper noun for pregnancy. A complete gestation period is a physiological process from conception to delivery. Throughout the process, the sperm inseminates the egg, becoming a fertilized egg that divides into about 100 blastocyst cells. The embryo implantation succeeds, develops, and grows until the final delivery. Every step in the middle that malfunctions may lead to pregnancy failure.

According to a *China Economic Weekly* survey, even for a married couple with no physical problems at all, there is a 40% chance that they will not be able to conceive within half a year and a 20% chance that they will not be able to conceive within a year or so. Relevant statistics show that among the various causes of infertility, separate male and female factors account for about 30% to 40%, couple factors for 20%, and the remaining 10% are unknown.

There are many causes of infertility. Generally, the main causes of male infertility are related to sperm quality, quantity, and sexual performance. It is worth mentioning that in recent years, the unqualified rate of semen quality has been increasing yearly. Studies of sperm counts in men have been going on for decades, and these studies share the finding that human sperm counts have been declining since the beginning of the 20th century, and so has the level of hormones such as testosterone in men.

In 2017, Hagai Levine of the Hebrew University of Jerusalem conducted an extensive data analysis. His team selected 185 studies from 1973 to 2011 and accurately analyzed the sperm counts of over 40,000 men from over 50 countries in North America and Europe. The results were surprising in that the sperm counts of men from North America, Europe, Australia, and New Zealand had fallen by 53% over the past 40 years.

In China, over time, the semen concentration and total sperm counts of Chinese men have experienced a significant decrease in the 14 years since 1995. W.H.O. has even lowered the standard for qualified semen twice. The *W.H.O. Laboratory Manual for the Examination and Processing of Human Semen* stipulates that the male sperm counts be adjusted from an average of 100 million per milliliter in 1970 to the current 15 million per milliliter.

The causes of women's infertility are more complex from a female perspective. For example, polycystic ovaries or premature ovarian failure can lead to ovulation disorders; blockage of fallopian tubes prevents eggs from combining with sperm; uterine diseases or autoimmunity impede fertilized eggs from implanting, etc. Even if a woman is impregnated, her hormone levels, physical condition, and stress during her pregnancy may cause the fetus to stop developing and the pregnancy to fail.

Among them, polycystic ovary syndrome is common among infertile patients. Patients with polycystic ovary syndrome are prone to follicle immaturity, persistent anovulation, androgen excess, and insulin resistance. Most of them will suffer from menstrual disorder, amenorrhea, infertility, hairiness, obesity, etc. And, for some, even when the cause is identified, the treatment takes a long time.

A.R.T. breeds an emerging market

Infertility is becoming a secret anguish. And there is no sign of it slowing down. Under such circumstances, Assisted Reproductive Technology (A.R.T.) has become inevitable. And it has generated a new business. From 2014 to 2018, the global auxiliary market expanded from US$ 20.4 billion to US$ 24.8 billion, with a Compound Annual Growth Rate (CAGR) of 5.1%.

The A.R.T. market size of China increased from US$ 2.3 billion to US$ 3.8 billion, with a CAGR of 13.6%; that of the U.S. grew from US$ 2.9 billion to US$ 3.7 billion, with a CAGR of 6.6%. It is estimated that from 2018 to 2023, the global A.R.T. market is expected to expand from US$ 24.8 billion to US$ 31.7 billion, with a CAGR of 5.0%, the U.S. market from US$ 3.7 billion to US$ 4.9 billion, with a CAGR of 5.9%, and the Chinese market from US$ 3.8 billion to US$ 7.5 billion, with a CAGR of 14.5%. And the market penetration in China will continue to increase.

A.R.T. can be roughly divided into three categories: artificial insemination, gamete intrauterine transfer (G.I.U.T.), and in-vitro fertilization (IVF). Artificial insemination is a technique in which sperm is delivered non-coitally into the female reproductive tract to impregnate a woman; G.I.U.T. performs a laparoscopic or small abdominal incision to transfer the gametes (mature eggs and active sperm) directly into the ampulla or the uterine cavity of the fallopian tube so that natural insemination takes place in the normal fallopian tubes of the human body; IVF is an artificial method to fertilize the egg in vitro. When the early embryos mature, they are transplanted into the mother's uterus for development and delivery.

IVF is the mainstream choice for assisted reproduction and the key profit-making project for reproductive centers. It has the highest comprehensive pregnancy rate, about 40%-60%, and the overall impact of women on embryo quality is 80%. According to the comprehensive pregnancy rate statistics of the core A.R.T. evaluation indicators, the overall pregnancy rates for conventional drug treatment, artificial insemination, and IVF are 15%, 20%, and 40%-60%, respectively. The success rate of IVF is far higher than other technologies, so it is also the leading A.R.T. at present.

In addition to IVF, with the advent of the celibate society, as more and more single women refuse to get married, their fertility wishes have become more prominent. In western countries, the number of women who freeze their eggs continues to grow.

In 2012, the American Society for Reproductive Medicine (ASRM) officially removed the "experimental" label of egg freezing technology, and the clinical application of egg freezing was opened. In 2014, Facebook and Apple announced that their employees would receive egg freezing insurance for non-medical purposes as a corporate employee benefit. According to data released by the American Society for Assisted Reproductive Technology (S.A.R.T.), there were 10,936 frozen egg cases in the U.S. in 2017. And such cases are expected to increase by 25% annually in the upcoming years. The frozen egg market in European countries such as Belgium, Switzerland, and Spain keeps expanding.

It is worth mentioning that compared with female fertility protection, male fertility protection is more mature. Sperm cryopreservation is the leading method of male fertility preservation. Self-sperm cryopreservation is the most important fertility preservation measure in clinical practice. The cryopreservation of spermatogonia stem cells is still in the laboratory stage. In China, compared with the description in the *Basic Standards and Technical Specifications for Human Sperm Banks* issued by the former Ministry of Health: men can apply for semen preservation for the purpose of reproductive health care or sperm preservation for future reproduction regardless of their marital status. However, freezing eggs for single women does not comply with the relevant provisions of Chinese laws and regulations to delay childbirth.

Finally, as there are in modern society more infertile patients, homosexual couples, and families who have lost their only child, the controversy about surrogacy has intensified. Surrogacy refers to the act of implanting fertilized eggs into the uterus of a fertile woman (a surrogate) by means of modern medical techniques (A.R.T. and its derived technologies), who then completes the pregnancy and childbirth for others (the client).

Surrogacy, as a highly controversial but popular means of breeding human offspring, stirs up disputes because it involves technical, ethical, and legal issues.

It goes against the traditional definition of "mother" and turns "gestation" into a commodity that can be bought with money. Though surrogacy satisfies the desire of a married couple to have a family and is in line with ethics, it is bound to have an impact on traditional marriage ethics because it is not clear who the parents of the child are when they have to use donated sperms and eggs. In commercial surrogacy, renting the uterus as a reproductive tool and commodity also challenges people's traditional family views.

Therefore, while surrogacy can help infertile women realize their dream of becoming mothers, the choice of surrogate mothers, their privacy and rights, parent-child relationship, and whether the children can only have limited contact with the surrogate mothers are bound to pose new challenges. This also raises further serious social, legal, and ethical issues.

In addition, surrogate mothers must have a mature and healthy uterus and must be voluntary. However, as illegal surrogacy is aimed at high profits, there are inevitably major health problems.

The commercialization of surrogacy will lead surrogate mothers who suffer from tremendous life pressures and surrogacy agencies with no bottom line who seek maximum benefits to set aside the actual physical condition of the surrogate mothers and perform frequent pregnancies, multiple pregnancies, and pregnancy through coitus. This affects the surrogate children's health and increases the risk of gestational death and sequelae (an aftereffect of a disease, condition, or injury)of the surrogate mothers.

Indeed, the impact of surrogacy is not only limited to itself, but it terribly challenges marital ethics. Surrogacy provides a single individual with an opportunity to have a family independently, allowing single men to "have full custody" of a child through egg donation and surrogate mothers. There is no marriage involved, nor does it require a romantic relationship, so there will never be a fight over custody. However, all social and ethical issues, at the root, need to be restrained by sound systems and laws.

At present, the attitude of all social sectors towards surrogacy is fickle. With the needs of the development of the times and the continuous advancement of the rule of law in various countries, surrogacy in the future will face more disputes, either for or against. In fact, in the two-way role of legal cultural innovation and medical science and technology advancement, medical science and technology is the most fundamental driving force. At the same time, the law will eventually regulate and guide the development direction of medicine. Surrogacy is an inevitable predicament in modern society. It is precisely because it poses new challenges to many social areas that we should confront it with a rational and peaceful attitude.

Based on current trends, we can predict that by 2035, babies born through surrogacy around the world will have at least tripled, and the primary means of surrogacy before that year will have still been through traditional, non-surrogate ways. But around the middle of the 21st century, human-assisted reproduction will go through a fundamental change from mother-dependent conception to in vitro fertilization and in vitro breeding. With the further maturity of gene editing and genetic recombination, more and more people will choose in vitro gene editing to have a baby instead of natural conception. Though this topic is facing bioethical challenges all over the world, it does not affect the development and application of the underground maternity industry chain in this regard.

Whether we accept it or not, human fertility will adopt the mode of industrial production in this century. Life science and technology development will continue to refresh the bioethical standards established by human society in the past and reconstruct the cognition of new bioethics.

5.4 When We Coexist with Cancer

Cancer is becoming a common and chronic disease that can be controlled.

According to the relevant data of the International Agency for Research on Cancer (I.A.R.C.), a subsidiary of the W.H.O., there were approximately 19.29 million new cancer cases in 2020, including 10.06 million males and 9.23 million females. One in five people worldwide will have cancer in their lifetime. Cancer's survival rate continues to increase with the growing number of cancer patients.

The New England Journal of Medicine has pinpointed that the number of cancer survivors has increased in the past 40 years. For example, the number of cancer survivors in the U.S. rose from 3.6 million in 1975 to 15.5 million in 2016. It is estimated that this number will have increased further to 26 million by 2040, most of whom are aged between 50 and 85.

From being afraid to talk about cancer to coexisting with it, cancer is changing from a death sentence in the past to a disease that can be lived with and does not have to be cured.

Cancer has become a common disease

All cancers begin in cells and undergo an evolution from emergence to expansion to metastasis. During that, gene mutation is the key to the development of cancer cells.

Mutations can happen by chance during cell division. When a cell mutates, it implies that some healthy cells in the human body no longer follow the body's instructions and are likely out of control. Mutations confer certain selective advantages to mutated cells over neighboring cells. When present in a group of genes (cancer driver genes), the mutated form affects the homeostatic development of a range of key cell functions.

This is also why cancer, a disease with many varieties that are difficult and expensive to treat, is closely related to age. After all, the older a person is, as time goes by, the easier genes mutate and trigger cancer under the influence of environmental and personal behavioral factors. On this basis, as the aging population arrives, the number of cancer patients will inevitably continue to expand.

And as the population ages, cancer is increasingly linked to young people. Today, the younger ages of cancer patients have become a widely accepted conclusion in the medical community, and cancer is approaching younger age groups without being noticed.

For example, in February 2020, a study involving researchers from the International Agency for Research on Cancer (I.A.R.C.) compared and analyzed nearly 1.85 million cases of young cancer patients from 41 countries in Asia, Europe, Africa, South and North America, and Oceania. It found that among the 15-to-39-year-olds, cancer rates were on the rise in 23 of the 41 countries during the study period, including China.

In China, excluding melanoma, the incidence of cancer in young men has increased by about 0.75% per year and in young women by about 1.82% per year. Cancer incidence remains stable in 16 countries; only two countries experience a smaller incidence. Among the younger population, thyroid cancer, testicular cancer, and three obesity-related cancers, including rectal cancer, breast cancer, and kidney cancer, have increased yearly.

The incidence of thyroid cancer increased significantly in 33 countries, of which South Korea had the most significant annual growth rate of 26.30% in men and 21.28% in women. For testicular cancer, the countries with the larger increase in incidence were located in Asia, and Kuwait had the greatest (10.47%). The incidence of breast cancer in women is climbing in most countries, mainly in Western and Eastern Europe and Asia.

For another example, in December 2020, a study published in *J.A.M.A. Network Open*, a sub-issue of the *Journal of the American Medical Association* (*J.A.M.A.*), once again confirmed the troubling trend of the younger age of cancer patients. It found that in 1973, there were 57.2 cancer cases in every 100,000 adolescents and young adults; in 2015, that number grew to 74.2. Between 1973 and 2015, cancer incidence in adolescents and young adults rose by 29.6%. In addition, women were generally more prone to cancer than men. Cancer occurs not only in younger people but also among women. More women than men were diagnosed with cancer in the 20–35 age range, reversing the numbers for the 15-19 age group. Modern medicine believes that environmental factors are one of the main carcinogenic factors. With the increasingly fierce contradiction between environmental protection and economic development, people have become deeply aware of the adverse effects of air pollution, smoking, and other environmental factors on physical health. For example, lung cancer is one of the most common cancers in the world, and its morbidity and mortality rates are increasing yearly.

Dietary factors often lead to gastrointestinal cancers. Smoked, roasted, and fried foods, preservatives, and additives added to fast food are all possible carcinogenic factors. As people pick up the pace of life, the proportion of fast food in the daily diet of young and middle-aged groups has gradually increased. An unhealthy diet can significantly increase the risk of cancer. In addition, foods high in calories and cholesterol may also raise the risk of cancer, while eating more vegetables and fruits can reduce that.

In addition, psychosocial factors are more likely to become one of the critical factors leading to cancer in younger people. Usually, the human body's immunologic surveillance can quickly identify cancer cells and inhibit or kill them.

However, factors such as excessive work pressure, psychological burdens, and disharmony in marital relationships can trigger a series of negative emotions, such as anxiety, irritability, pessimism, and disappointment. These adverse social psychological factors will cause dysfunction of a person's endocrine, nervous, and immune systems and further increase the likelihood of carcinogenesis.

As a result, the aging population, together with various carcinogenic factors in the development of modern society, makes cancer a common disease today, and there are more and more cancer patients around us.

Cancer has become a chronic disease

In fact, as early as 2006, the W.H.O. officially included cancer in the category of chronic diseases. In terms of its definition, chronic diseases are common non-communicable diseases, such as hypertension, hyperglycemia, hyperlipidemia, and hyperuricemia. Cancer, as one of the chronic diseases, shares the common characteristics of being non-infectious, having a slow onset, long course, and often recurring.

From the perspective of cancer pathogenesis, the occurrence of cancer results from a long period of evolution in the human body. Cancer development goes through a battle with the immune system even after cancer cells mutate. Moreover, cancer cells that escape the immune system's attack remain in the tissue where they have developed.

For example, superficial tumors, such as bladder linings or breast ducts, are called carcinoma in situ. Cancer cells expand and divide to create more cells and eventually grow a tumor. Tumors may contain millions of cancer cells. All body tissues have a membrane that holds the cells within the tissue. When cancer cells break through this membrane, they become invasive carcinoma.

As the tumor grows larger, its center moves further and further away from the blood vessels in the area where it grew. As a result, there is less and less oxygen and nutrients in the tumor center. Cancer cells cannot live without oxygen and nutrients like all healthy cells. Consequently, cancer cells send out signals, a.k.a. angiogenic factors, to encourage new blood vessels to grow into the tumor.

Once cancer can stimulate blood vessel growth, it becomes bigger and faster and then stimulates the growth of hundreds of new capillaries to bring in nutrients and oxygen again. In addition, a tumor can take up so much space in the body that it puts pressure on surrounding structures, including random expansion from where it started.

This is the ultimate cancer, a.k.a. infiltrating carcinoma, which suggests that the cancer cells have invaded and infiltrated deeper from where they occurred. The prolonged onset of cancer has given it the characteristics of a chronic disease.

From the perspective of cancer treatment, as early as 1981, the W.H.O. proposed that cancer be a chronic disease. One-third of cancers can be prevented, 1/3 can be cured if detected, diagnosed, and treated early, and 1/3, though incurable, can be controlled via proper treatment to maintain a better quality of life, thereby prolonging their survival.

In terms of curability, it takes at least three years from the emergence of cancer cells to the growth of a cancer mass with a diameter of 1 cm. The slow growth process gives people ample time to detect, diagnose, and treat it early, which is the secondary prevention of cancer. According to 2014 statistics on cancer by the American Cancer Society (A.C.S.), cancer mortality has steadily declined, with an overall drop of 20%, due to active prevention, early detection, and standardized treatment.

Though it is incurable for the remaining one-third of advanced cancer patients, with several great leaps in medical treatment and the emergence of more and more anti-cancer methods such as chemotherapy, targeted therapy, and immunotherapy, the survival rate of cancer patients has been dramatically improved. For example, the five-year survival rate for patients with chronic myeloid leukemia has increased to 90% from 30% 15 years ago. The patient can live nearly 20 years longer if the medication is taken in time.

Another example is early-stage lung cancer. After surgical resection, its five-year survival rate exceeds 90%, and its ten-year survival rate is also high. In the 1980s and 1990s, the median survival of advanced lung cancer in China was no more than ten months. The medical peaks we continue to conquer have gradually transformed more and more cancers into chronic diseases.

The post-cancer era

Since cancer has gradually become a common and chronic disease, how to prevent and coexist with it is a problem that people need to rethink.

As mentioned above, 1/3 of cancers are preventable as a chronic disease—over 30% of cancer could be avoided through a healthy lifestyle such as not smoking, keeping a healthy diet, maintaining physical activity, and strictly limiting alcohol consumption. However, while science and technology provide a more efficient and convenient lifestyle, they also make people's lives more irregular and uncontrolled.

The World Cancer Report 2014 pointed out that although the medical community has long clearly identified many risk factors for cancer, such as smoking, alcohol abuse, unhealthy diets, obesity, lack of exercise, and so on, these problems still exist in the low- to medium-income countries. In contrast, developed countries have witnessed dramatic declines in cancer incidence and mortality in recent years due to the active promotion of healthy lifestyles.

From the perspective of coexistence with cancer, the top two of the four chronic diseases with the highest mortality rate in the world are cancer (28.1%) and cardiovascular and cerebrovascular diseases (27.1%). It is easy to see that the mortality rate of cardiovascular disease is similar to that of cancer. However most people take cardiovascular disease calmly, but cancer feels like a death sentence to them. The fear of cancer far exceeds other diseases, and the root of such fear is that the public knows little of and misunderstands cancer.

Therefore, many over-treatments have happened under the ignorance and fear of cancer. In July 2017, the *New England Journal of Medicin* published a prospective clinical study on prostatectomy and follow-up observations of early-stage prostate cancer. After nearly 20 years of observations, the researchers found that the surgery group did not significantly reduce all causes of prostate cancer mortality compared with the control group.

61.3% of the patients in the surgery group died, while 66.8% in the control group died (HR 0.84; P=0.06); 7.4% of the deaths in the surgery group were attributable to prostate cancer or treatment, while the number of the control group was 11.4% (HR 0.63; P=0.06). That said, surgery did not significantly reduce the chance of death. However, in treating tumors, many people believe that the operation to remove tumors should be "grand and comprehensive."

In fact, cancer patients are in poor physical condition, and surgery, as a treatment method, cannot avoid surgical failure, post-op complications, and poor quality of life during the recovery. Especially for patients with advanced cancer, surgery is obviously not the best choice when the evaluation concludes that surgery helps little to improve the patient's quality of life and slow the progression of the disease.

Psychologically, it is no embarrassment to admit having cancer, actively treat it, take appropriate measures to control it or cure it, build a new balance with it, and survive for decades with it present. Coexisting with cancer requires stopping excessive treatment and moving towards appropriate therapies. It is never about the size of the incision. We should loosen the absolutist stance of "tumor-free" survival and truly embrace "tumor-bearing" survival.

I can foresee that by 2035, the medical community will have initiated a discussion on the condition of cancer and sought to redefine the criteria of cancer treatment success, which will no longer be the shrinkage or disappearance of tumor tissue in the absolute sense, but the prolongation of survival and the improvement of the quality of life. Society's recognition of cancer will change from the "afraid to talk about it" to coexisting with it. And the removal of the tumor is no longer the criterion for a full recovery but when the body reaches a state of balance and harmony.

Cancer-promoting and tumor-suppressing genes coexist in the human body. With a rational understanding of the fear of cancer and the search for more tumor-promoting gene inhibitory drugs and tumor-suppressing gene activation methods, our mindset will change from eradicating and fighting cancer to treating and living with it.

5.5 The Future Trend of Artificial Meat

Humans will never give up eating meat. As food biotechnology advances, artificial meat has been invented to meet people's diverse needs for meat. In the past few years, the popularity of the artificial meat industry has been evident to all, and the favor of large capital—investors like Bill Gates and companies like Cargill and Tyson have put tens of millions of dollars in related companies—has promoted the rapid development of the artificial meat market.

Many start-ups have risen rapidly, launching the world's first vegan meat pie, artificial meat burgers, cell-cultured steak, chicken, etc. Traditional food giants such as K.F.C., Starbucks, Burger King, and Nestlé have also entered this industry, launching artificial meat sandwiches, vegan chicken nuggets with vegetable protein, and other products through cooperative or independent R&D. The popularity of these products once boosted the popularity of the idea of artificial meat in the secondary market. It is predicted that with the continuous exploration of life science and technology and the continuous maturity of synthetic food technology, it is inevitable that artificial foods will continue to replace the current natural foods.

Plant meat and protein meat

According to the different raw materials and processing techniques, artificial meat is divided into two categories: plant and cellular. Between them, plant meat refers to the use of vegetable protein of soybeans, peas, and other plants to produce and process foods similar to animal meat in food texture, taste, or appearance through special processes, such as shredded dried tofu, vegan meat, vegan chicken, fake meat for vegetarian monks, and many other soy products.

It is worth mentioning that the most significant difference between artificial plant meat and traditional vegan meat, which has long been in the domestic market, lies in the raw materials and processing techniques used. The two most essential links in producing artificial plant meat are the acquisition of soybean and pea protein and the R&D of core technologies such as synthesizing and processing artificial plant meat.

Specifically, traditional vegan meat primarily uses soybeans and tofu as the main raw materials. In most cases, no deep processing is performed to extract vegetable protein. In the later stage, only the physical process of thermal processing is required to build a meat-like food texture. At the same time, artificial plant meat uses plant protein separated from soybeans and peas as raw materials. Its subsequent production process is more complicated, requiring advanced synthetic biotechnology and a series of processes such as fermentation and extrusion.

Compared with cellular meat, at this point in time, plant meat is the most critical commercialization direction of artificial meat. The more well-known companies in the market, such as Beyond Meat, Impossible Food, Zhen Meat, and Starfield, are representatives of the plant meat field. For example, the extraction of soy hemoglobin from Impossible Foods' plant-based meatloaf is a special technique—the oxygenated iron compound present in all living cells makes meat red and sells for US$ 12 apiece. Impossible Foods has partnered with 1,400 burger shops in the U.S., of which the high-end burger chain Umami Burger has sold more than 200,000 burgers with it.

Compared to plant meat, cellular meat seems to resemble real meat better. Cellular meat is also called animal meat. It extracts totipotent (a single cell that can give rise to a new organism) stem cells or muscle cells from animals and cultures them in a nutrient solution to grow through cell proliferation and form tissue-like substances. As assumed by experts in the field of cellular agriculture, this kind of meat "grown" in the laboratory by extracting animal cells is comparable to real meat in terms of appearance, taste, and nutrients.

In fact, as early as the early 1990s, artificial meat was one of the research projects funded by NASA. Americans tried to use cellular meat technology to solve the food problem of space travel. It wasn't until 2013 that Dutch biologist Mark Post made the world's first cellular meat burger from the lab at the cost of US$ 325,000. It has been five years since the first piece of cellular meat was made, but the price of a pound of artificial chicken meat at Memphis Meats, an American artificial meat manufacturer, is still as high as US$ 9,000. In comparison, boneless chicken breasts cost about US$ 3.22 per pound to produce in the U.S., which is one of the reasons why artificial cellular meat has not yet hit the market.

Though artificial meat remains highly expensive, it is almost inevitable that technology will lower the cost of cellular meat. For example, Israeli cellular meat company Future Meat Technologies (F.M.T.) is trying to overcome the cost dilemma by using patented technology for culture medium filtration regeneration. In 2019, the price of a pound of chicken cultured in the F.M.T. lab was US$ 150. After over a year of technical research, it dropped to US$ 3.90.

Recently, F.M.T. announced its intermediate pilot plant in Rehovot, Israel, has been completed. It has become one of the few companies in the industry that uses culture medium filtration regeneration technology to achieve mass production. Its C.E.O. Rom Kshuk stated his expectation to reduce costs to less than US$ 2 in the next 12–18 months. He compared the lowered cost of artificial meat to buying a Tesla Model X at US$ 129.

There is no doubt that the cellular laboratory meat can be scaled up once the technical bottleneck is broken and will set off a storm in the artificial meat market.

The inevitable future of food

With the continuous exploration of life science and technology and the continuous maturity of synthetic food technology, artificial food inevitably continues to replace the current natural food.

This is because, in terms of the safety of artificial meat that some people are questioning, the existing artificial meat is as safe as other ordinary processed foods on the market. In fact, as long as the raw and auxiliary materials and food additives used in production are up to the standards, cross-contamination is avoided in the production, sampling inspection is well performed before the products are shipped out of the factory, and supervision is in place during the circulation, the quality and safety of artificial meat can be ensured.

In addition to ensuring safety, artificial food can also retain the beneficial elements that our human body needs, and eliminate some harmful and ineffective food elements, which may help prolong people's lifespan. Judging from the plant meat on the market, the official website of Beyond Meat promotes its products by claiming they have the same protein content as meat or even higher, less saturated fatty acids, and zero cholesterol.

For example, the W.H.O., the Chinese Nutrition Society, and the American Heart Association all recommend that the energy supply ratio of saturated fatty acids be controlled within 10%. The pork, beef, and mutton we eat have higher saturated fatty acid content while replacing saturated fatty acids with unsaturated fatty acids is conducive to improving dyslipidemia.

Based on this, during the simulation of the fat content of real meat, the content of saturated fatty acids in plant meat can be controlled by properly arranging the ratio of various vegetable oils and increasing the content of unsaturated fatty acids. Therefore, the nutrition of plant meat is almost completely higher than that of ordinary meat. This further caters to the people's needs and consumption concepts for health, quality, and individuality.

In addition, from a macro level, artificial meat can effectively reduce the negative impact on the environment and is more in line with the present environmental protection philosophy. Traditional animal husbandry is the primary source of two major greenhouse gases (methane and nitrous oxide). It generates more greenhouse gases than cars, trucks, planes, trains, and ships combined, directly triggering global warming.

In addition, the development of traditional animal husbandry will consume great natural resources such as land, crops, and water, resulting in waste of resources. In recent years, as people pay more heed to environmental protection, all walks of life have introduced environmental, social, and governance (E.S.G.) evaluation standards. In this context, the transformation of traditional animal husbandry is inevitable, and the emergence of artificial meat is a necessary part of such a transformation.

The prospectus of Beyond Meat shows that when artificial meat replaces common edible meat, there will be 90% less greenhouse gas emissions, 99% less use of water resources, 93% less use of land, and 46% less use of energy resources. According to data released by the Food and Agriculture Organization (F.A.O.) of the U.N., traditional meat production accounts for 18% of greenhouse gas emissions, 30% of land use, and 8% of water and energy consumption.

Despite the absence of a systematic assessment of the impact of artificial meat on the environment at the moment, it has at least reduced resource consumption and greenhouse gas emissions during its production, as well as the environmental pollution caused by veterinary drugs used in the raising the livestock.

Artificial meat begins high and ends low

In recent years, the concept of artificial meat has become extremely popular. With the help of massive capital, plant meat companies have been registered and opened one after another, and some have continued to set new financing records. Contrary to the capital fever, many plant meat products are short-lived when the current core technology and implementation scenarios are not yet clear.

Affected by the COVID-19 pandemic and the sales of a B-end retail business, the leading company Beyond Meat has experienced increasing losses in recent quarters; in the C-end consumer market, the poor consumption of it is an embarrassment. At Starbucks in China, the price of Classic Lasagna with plant-based beef has been marked down from the original RMB 69 to RMB 49. On the whole, Starbucks' vegan meat series, which were generally priced at RMB 50–60 at the beginning, have been marked down to RMB 30–40.

From the concept's popularity to the harsh reality, it takes time for the vegan meat that opens high and ends low to bounce back. Generally, the food area has powerful traditional strength and solidified thinking. While most of the innovations in other areas are widely accepted, people always pay more careful scrutiny to the innovation of food ingredients. Though foreign companies have begun to seize the Chinese artificial meat market, artificial meat has not been widely recognized by Chinese consumers. There is limited acceptance and popularity of artificial meat in China.

The report *China's Plant Meat Market Insights* revealed the essential characteristics of the Chinese artificial meat consumer groups: most of them reside in first-tier cities, are aged between 30 and 40, are more receptive to novelties, pursue a quality lifestyle, attach great importance to health management, and can afford higher-priced food. This implies that in the Chinese market, it will take more time for artificial meat to have regular consumption in the meat market.

Moreover, for most consumers, price is the most detrimental factor. *Nanfang Daily* once disclosed a set of data: in the U.S., the price of one kg of processed meat is US$ 7, while the same amount of plant meat costs US$ 15. In the American chain Walmart, the final retail price of beef burgers produced by food factories is currently US$ 2.80/lb, while Beyond Meat's plant-meat burgers are sold at US$ 6.25/lb.

Omnipork, the first plant meat brand to enter the Chinese market, sells its plant meat for about RMB 60 per kilogram, while the cheapest pork on an e-commerce platform of fresh food is about RMB 50 per kilogram. Such a price obviously does not look attractive to Chinese consumers. Most respondents who have purchased plant meat complained that "It does not taste good."

Regarding food safety, there are currently no national, local, industry, or group standards for artificial meat. Most companies formulate their standards or produce them regarding foreign standards, which raises doubts in the market. At present, there is no perfect supply chain or perfect industrial chain for artificial meat in China. Basically, it is mainly import and cooperation. In addition to well-known large companies with strong credibility to endorse themselves, other companies who join the artificial meat race shortly will likely face doubts and poor recognition from Chinese consumers.

In general, plant meat is still in its early stages of development in China, and significant capital is needed for product R&D and supply chain construction. The production of plant meat can only be recognized by the market if it can significantly increase its production capacity, effectively reduce costs and prices, and cater to the taste of Chinese consumers. This undoubtedly makes higher requirements for the technical level of enterprises.

Artificial meat must be an opportunity for future food. As a consumer market that has just started, artificial meat still needs the participation and efforts of all parties, including the gradual education and cognition of consumers, the endorsement of chain catering companies, the promotion of market-oriented products, and the continuous iteration of technology and production plans by artificial meat startups. As the harm caused by environmental pollution to natural food continues to increase, people will become more aware of the benefits of artificial food. It is foreseeable that by around 2035, some developed countries will have had a considerable amount of artificial food to replace natural food. By the middle of the 21st century, more genetically modified and artificial foods with gene therapy will enter the supermarket. People will continue to accept genetically modified foods as they learn more about genetic engineering.

CHAPTER 6

Questions and Considerations on Ethical Values

THE HIGHLY ADVANCED INTERNET TECHNOLOGY HAS INSPIRED MORE AND more digital devices. Various digital devices such as smartphones, tablet PCs, and smart watches are increasingly penetrating people's lives, taking them to an unprecedentedly thriving information age. However, while digital technology has reshaped social concepts and enabled more efficient access to information, it has also brought more challenges.

The information created by the media and the online traffic screams the great slogans of the post-industrial era, advocating an exquisite life and individuality, and coaxing people into showing off their wealth; in the meantime, based on the world's situation, such as class solidification, consumption downgrades, and competition over family background, it ignites public anxiety. As an important watershed in the history of human development, the COVID-19 pandemic has profoundly changed our way of thinking and value identification, pushing us into a vacuum of ethical values.

Where there is the chaos of life, the disintegration of beliefs, and the at-a-loss of morality, the humanities are probably what only can console the human soul. The essence of humanities is a humanistic spirit, a culture different from science. The humanities don't teach people how to succeed but how to question success. A country's progress is reflected in the development of economy and science and technology, but also the improvement of humanistic quality and the level of civilization of social governance. Taking kindness as beauty is what makes us human beings.

6.1 Artificial Intelligence Challenges Man-Machine Boundaries

Under the inevitable trend of artificial intelligence (A.I.), A.I.'s regulatory challenges and ethical dilemmas have become a global problem. From AI's exposing nudity via "one-click undressing" with the help of a neural network to the continuous new inventions of sex robots and their commercial application, the development of A.I. has exacerbated social anxiety. In addition to worries about future ethics and the fear of unknown future social changes, what truly shakes human beings is the new challenge A.I. brings to human existence.

In the digital age, while the total amount of information we create is accumulated in geometric progression, human beings' spiritual existence and evolution have far exceeded the load our physical body can bear. Under such circumstances, how can we continue our adaptability and survive in this new world we build?

Highly developed robotics frees human beings from manual labor, and the continuous breakthroughs in brain-computer interface studies allow us to glimpse the possibility of future robots. The efficiency of human brain operations will be significantly improved, and even higher-level collective cooperation will be accomplished. By then, will humans still dominate the world? What is the truth of survival?

The technological fantasy of artificial intelligence

Whether it is weak A.I. or strong A.I., behind these technologies, there is still the physical image of the soul, the brain, and the first and foremost of technological fantasies must come from people and human nature.

The brain is the most unique organ of human beings. If a person's kidney and a pig's kidney are shown together, most people cannot distinguish them by the shape. However, if it is the brain, almost everyone can tell which is which.

Though the human brain looks like a large chunk of tofu carved into the shape of a walnut kernel, its essence is a network composed of neurons. And the neural networks in A.I. are constructed by mimicking the human brain. By orders of magnitude, the scientific community commonly believes that there are 100 billion neurons in the human brain. If it takes one second to count one neuron, it will take 3,100 years to count them all.

Each neuron casts a significant number of nerve fibers in all directions, and the cell body in the center receives whatever the fibers deliver. Most dendrites are responsible for obtaining and transmitting information among these nerve fibers, while only one axon (with branches) outputs information. When the dendrites receive information greater than the excitation threshold, the entire neuron bursts out with a short but undeniable action potential like a light bulb. Such potential travels along the cell membrane almost instantaneously throughout the neuron—including the nerve fiber ends far from the cell body.

Subsequently, the terminal structure called the synapse between the last neuron's axon and the next neuron's dendrite is activated by electrical signals, and the synapse immediately releases the neurotransmitter to transmit information between two neurons. According to its different types, it can either excite or inhibit the next neuron.

Neurons make up the basic structure of the human brain, including the cerebrum, which processes most of the thinking, the cerebellum, which coordinates movement, and the brainstem that connects them.

The brainstem connects the cerebrum, cerebellum, and spinal cord, through which nearly all neural projections between the brain and the body pass. In addition, the brainstem regulates essential life activities such as breathing, body temperature, and swallowing, and even the conscious actions of the brain need to be maintained by its reticular activating system (R.A.S.). Therefore, the brainstem is believed to be the most vulnerable vital part of the human body. Once damaged, it is instant death.

The structure of the cerebrum is more complex. The wrinkled surface we see is the folded and curled cerebral cortex that rapidly expands. Different parts of the cortex have different functional divisions. Beneath the cortex are the thalamus, amygdala, striatum, globus pallidus, and other oddly named nuclei. Modern science believes that the human cerebral cortex is the most developed organ that thinks and dominates all body activities and regulates the balance between the body and the surrounding environment. Therefore, the cerebral cortex is the material basis for advanced neural activities. Our present brains have evolved over millions of years, thus far more developed than earlier human brains.

Questions on the thought of human evolution

When *Sahelanthropus tchadensis* roamed in Africa seven million years ago, the cerebra in their cranial cavities were not fundamentally different from those of other animals. Millions of years later, when the Homo sapiens of Olduvai Gorge clumsily hammered out what might have been the earliest stone tools, their brains, not much more robust than those of chimpanzees, did not display astonishing intelligence.

During the following evolution, the Hominidae strengthened their ability to use and make tools. Their brains developed steadily, but something seemed to be something missing that suppressed their talent in the magnificent gene pool of nature. About 200,000 years ago, the brain of modern developed by leaps and bounds, and the contact cortex, which matters little to direct survival, especially the frontal lobe, experienced a dramatic surge, and led to high energy consumption (the human brain accounts for only about 2% of body weight, but consumes 20% of energy) and painful childbirth. But the result of paying these costs is that for the first time, the brain has so many neurons to perform deep abstract processing, sorting, and storing of various information.

Next, declarative memory and language appeared. Humans can summarize and extract abstract general concepts from specific and objective things and can accurately describe, communicate, and even learn them through language. Moreover, with the help of the change of thinking patterns brought about by language, human beings have acquired the ability of imagination.

The famous science fiction writer Itōu Keikaku describes in his novel *Genocidal Organs* that language is an organ in the brain by nature. But because of the advent of this brain structure, the developmental speed of human beings immediately accelerated explosively. Human beings evolved from naked apes in the corner of East Africa to a super ecological invasive species that spread worldwide.

Next, an imagined community based on language emerged, and human social behavior went beyond the tribal level of primate instinct and became larger and more complex. With the invention of writing, the earliest civilizations and city-states were born in Mesopotamia in Western Asia.

Another unique ability, working memory, enables humans to make plans and execute them step-by-step, which has immeasurable significance for human development. Patients with schizophrenia perform significantly worse than average people in this matter, which may be one of the reasons for their cognitive and behavioral disorders. On top of these abstract cognitive abilities, the human brain has one more scarce ability – self-cognition.

Like Socrates's timeless saying "know yourself," engraved on the stone foundation of the ancient temple of Babylon, self-awareness is not necessary for general decision-making tasks nor entirely associated with intelligence. But it is this ability that makes humans realize their existence and start to question: Who am I? Where am I from? Where am I going? And these three questions run through thousands of years of human philosophical thinking.

There is no doubt that no matter how technology or A.I. develops, it cannot escape the underlying and core logic of human thought, and this is the source of our anxiety in the face of the rapid development of A.I.

Redefine the man–machine boundary

In 2020, when the world fought against the COVID-19 pandemic, A.I. responded quickly in fields such as medical care, urban governance, industry, and contactless services. It has played a vital role in pandemic prevention and control, improving the overall efficiency of the fight against it. The unprecedentedly close integration of A.I. and industry has once again verified the actual value of A.I. to society as an important driving force for a new round of technological revolution and industrial transformation.

In terms of application, thanks to the rapid development of computer vision, image recognition, natural language processing, and other technologies, A.I. has widely penetrated into many vertical fields, cutting into different scenarios and applications and providing products and solutions, and its product forms are diversifying.

The COVID-19 pandemic has become a touchstone for A.I. During the pandemic, A.I. companies are no longer the bystanders as in the past but play critical roles, thereby improving the overall efficiency of the fight against the pandemic. In terms of medical treatment, A.I. realizes image recognition, improves medical efficiency, and performs medical screening to help new drug R&D. During the pandemic, A.I. technology has also promoted the development of remote consultation and online popularization of medical information, enabling people to access medical resources more efficiently and faster.

After the pandemic, there is no longer a pure traditional industry in the world because every industry has more or less started digitization. Affected by risk factors such as the difficulty of hiring employees, increased costs, and labor infections during the pandemic, the manufacturing, and service industries are accelerating the process of man-machine integration and further transforming into intelligent manufacturing and services. The pandemic has opened a new window and rich opportunities for practice to develop A.I., making the world of ubiquitous intelligence come true faster.

With the continuous development of technology, algorithms, scenarios, and talents, A.I. is infiltrating various fields, and its value has been verified in the fields of industry, medical care, and cities. Undoubtedly, in the future, more industries will be innovatively integrated with intelligent technology, and more new business forms and models will be born.

Under such circumstances, A.I. will replace most manual work. In various fields of human life and work, such as literary creation, intelligent driving, construction, investment and wealth management, social governance, and intelligent manufacturing, it will be a common phenomenon and a long-term trend that A.I. continues to replace human labor.

A.I., under the blessing of modern science, holds extraordinary powers that were once unimaginable to human beings. What have we become when we accept and adapt to these fantastic powers? How should the boundaries between humans and machines be redefined? Though many thinkers since the time of Descartes have wondered about the answer to these questions, the rapid changes in modern technology have thrown these questions directly to the general public in a more impactful way.

In a sense, when we are more and more closely connected with machines, we hand over the memory of the road to navigation and the memory of knowledge to the chip, and even our physiological needs and spiritual needs to sex robots. Therefore, behind the more convenient and efficient lifestyle that seems to be advancing continuously, the uniqueness of being a human has also suffered an irreversible degeneration with the assistance of machinery. The more we can do with technology, the less we can live without it.

As far as this threat may seem, ignoring it is genuinely terrifying. The emergence of A.I. has undoubtedly enabled us to accomplish many previously unimaginable tasks. The living conditions of human beings have been obviously changed, but when this change extends from the outside to the inside and shakes the way humans exist at the individual level, what we have to think about perhaps is no longer how to change the world, but how to embrace a gradually mechanized world.

Under the challenge of A.I., human beings will definitely rethink the division of labor and boundaries between humans and machines in the new world and the position of human beings. Obviously, the technology industry needs to shift from the current technology-centric model to the technology-humanities collaboration model. The R&D of A.I. needs to widely absorb the thinking and concerns of people from different races, genders, cultures, socioeconomic classes, and different fields.

It is foreseeable that with the continuous maturity and improvement of A.I. and robotics, by 2035 or so, 50% of the existing jobs in human society will have been replaced by robots. By the middle of the 22nd century, robots will have been able to perform 90% of human society's work. At that time, robots will be able to think independently, discuss and consider topics of philosophy and life together with human society.

6.2 Machine Companions Reshape Marriage Ethics

The rise of A.I. continues to reshape how people envision the future. And machine companions, as the most extensive field of future intelligent robot development, have been increasingly involved in people's lives. They play the role of assistants, friends, partners, and even family. Among the many types of machine companions, sex robots have been receiving continuous attention.

From celibacy to the difficulty of avoiding needs

In terms of needs, being single is becoming the "ism" of modern people.

Statistics show the number of marriages in the U.K. has dropped to the lowest level in the past 150 years; the unmarried rate of young men aged 30-34 in Japan is 47.1%, and that of young women is 32%; in Stockholm, capital of Sweden, such ratio is as high as 60%. About 50.2% of Americans over 16 remain single, that is 124.6 million people. Sixty years ago, in the 1950s, the marriage rate for adults in the U.S. was as high as 70%. As a populous nation, the population of singles in China is even greater. According to the recent Seventh National Census data released, the single adult population in China has reached 240 million. Among them, more than 77 million people are single and living alone.

Chinese sociologist Li Yinhe believes that a single society first means the rapid rise of individualism, that marriage has changed from a universal value to a purely individual choice, and the concept of family and familialism are declining. Throughout history, human life and livelihoods have generally involved three primary structures, which, from the inside out, are the central family, the extended family, and the local community of families. As the basic unit of society, the family's status is unchallengeable, and marriage, the starting point of a new family, is in the center of the spotlight.

But now, services provided by local governments and agencies have replaced the family responsibilities in the past, including food and clothing, health care, education, and housing. A traditional family's indispensable role in caring for family members is gradually being replaced by thriving state and market forces. As the family is no longer necessary for individual survival, a series of family changes and marriages begin to happen.

In this context, sexual needs are unavoidable. According to *Business Insider*, since the COVID-19 pandemic, sales of the world's first A.I. sex robot Harmony have surged, even though it is priced as high as US$ 12,000. In 2019, futurist Dr. Ian Pearson published a predictive report on the future of sex. He predicts that around 2050, human-robot sex will become popular, and robots may even replace human sexual partners.

Dr. Pearson's prediction seems to be coming true. As the cost of sex robots continues to drop and their functions continue to improve, sex robots are no longer beyond reach. For instance, Harmony 2.0 has become more like a real companion. It has richer facial expressions, more flexible limbs, and more realistic body skin. Thanks to its built-in heater, it can also simulate actual body temperature.

In addition, Harmony 2.0 integrates Amazon's voice system, Alexa, so that it can analyze the sound information in time, quickly give accurate feedback, and make simple responses to various topics. Meanwhile, it is also equipped with an intelligent software system, which can store and memorize past chats to determine partners' habits and preferences. That is to say, Harmony 2.0 will have a deeper and deeper understanding of the user after a long period of companionship. In the future, sex robots will become more and more diverse and sexier and sexier.

Marriage under ethical challenge

The trend of a single society, together with the unavoidable needs, and the continuous advancement of technology, has brought sex robots to people's attention. The COVID-19 pandemic has created a demand for them. Data shows that Harmony's sales increased by at least 50% during the wide outbreak of COVID-19. And another sex doll company, Silicone Lovers, also stated that orders for sex robots have been pouring in since the pandemic outbreak.

However, with the development of sex robots and their market opening, human marriage is bound to be challenged by ethics. When sex robots enter human society, marriage must be the first thing they will change drastically. Marriage is not necessarily going to be canceled but must become a diversified existence.

When a sex robot can replace an actual human partner, the long stable symbiotic relationship between men and women will become a competitive relationship. Perhaps there will no longer be the concept of family because every family composed of husband and wife will become independent individuals in society. In this process, to pass on life, human beings will choose to buy sperm and eggs, and special personnel will carry out the surrogacy. The concept of human beings as the sum of social relations may no longer exist because the family in this era is each individual with the same social competitiveness and their artificial partners, which is somehow an ideal state.

Meanwhile, people's sexual desires will be significantly reduced because regardless of male or female, their artificial partners will absolutely obey the orders and can be highly customized. But sex, as uniquely human behavior, is diverse. Quite a few people in this world are into unconventional sexual behavior. It is still unknown whether sex robots will eventually damage human exploration and curiosity because of mechanical limitations.

Perhaps, for sex robots, while people gain the pleasure of being in control, they may also lose the pleasure of being out of control. People get a sense of absolute security—never abandoned, rejected, and left out, but at the same time, they reject the unease of solitude. Where there is demand, there is a market. Without a doubt, sex robots will happen and inevitably become part of the future sex industry. The infiltration of technology will also transform the sex industry, thereby affecting human sexual culture.

In addition to sex robots, virtual sex will also become mainstream. With the help of virtual reality equipment, couples far apart can have a remote sexual relationship with sex aids and change the scenes and characters according to their preference without the other party's knowledge to meet their own physical and mental needs. At that time, marriage will become a philosophical topic, and the present marriage system will be gradually ignored and eventually end.

6.3 Unresolved Privacy Conundrums

First, picture a daily situation: a news app on your smartphone that you use often pushes some ads, but since it does not affect your reading experience, you don't care much. Then, the ad content seems concerning as it frequently shows real estate sales openings in your city. You're uncomfortable because you realize your location is exposed. Next, it gets worse. The name of your community appears in the ad for second-hand apartment sales.

Let's picture another case: you keep receiving many text messages in the first two days of a shopping festival. The frequency is so high that they fill your screen. At the end of each text message, write To unsubscribe, please reply T. You are aware this will not work, and block the senders directly, leaving no chance for them. However, over time, the number of your text messages does not go down. You might think the telecom carriers are doing a poor job.

The above two cases are both imaginary and real. In the Internet Age, obtaining an individual's private information is easy because too many links leak privacy. Any platform that involves exchanging information, from matchmaking to takeaway delivery, from exams to housekeeping, from ticket purchase to insurance. Privacy will definitely be leaked when personal information is left in one of the above links. It's just a matter of time. What is frustrating is even though you know that your privacy will be leaked, you have no choice but to accept it. In the end, you can only hope that your information is too invaluable to be packaged and sold via extensive data integration.

The pandemic has catalyzed the digital revolution and accelerated the formation of historical turning points. Human society is marching from the physical world into the digital world, and the interconnection and digitization of all things have become a trend. Statistics show that the data produced by humans in the past few years accounted for 95% of human beings' entire historical data volume. In other words, the era of big data has truly arrived. Meanwhile, privacy issues have gradually come into focus.

During the pandemic, it can be seen from the launch of digital monitoring systems such as health codes that privacy has been intertwined in our daily lives. Whether it is the Internet of Things or intelligent media brought by 5G, they are both based on big data, and this data naturally contains massive amounts of user privacy. We can even believe that the higher the level of media intelligence, the more serious the violation of personal privacy rights. And the previous concept that all privacy is private only is neither realistic nor desirable in the era of big data. While the intelligent system serves human beings, it also poses an invisible threat of unprecedented privacy crisis to people's lives.

New features of data privacy in the era of big data

In 2019, the world ushered in the first year of 5G. Governments have successively issued 5G commercial licenses. In 2020, 5G entered a period of rapid development, which inevitably led to a substantial increase in uplink data traffic so that data of greater magnitude, variety, and timeliness came true.

Big data are mainly characterized by its ultra-large-scale and strong instantaneity. The ultra-large-scale can satisfy the ultra-high connection density. According to application requirements, the Internet of Everything will continue to produce, transmit, analyze, and consume data, thus quickly increasing the amount of data in the era of big data in terms of data generation subjects and data types. Under the support of 5G technology, the strong instantaneity makes it possible to render data services with millisecond-level low latency and present a more distinct real-time characteristic.

There is no doubt that the characteristics of data in the era of big data will react upon and profoundly impact personal information and private data.

Primarily, in the era of big data, the density of private data has decreased while its number has increased. The data in the age of big data are characterized by its large scale and strong real-time. The quantity, type, unstructured degree of data, frequency, instantaneity, and granularity of data collection have been greatly improved. The development of the digital economy will further unleash more potential in the era of data processing technology.

The extensive data collection supported by 5G technology involves more personal and private information, though the proportion of this information in the overall information is reduced. However, there will be a substantial increase in absolute volume. In terms of smart city construction, extensive data collection focuses more on the movement trajectories of people and vehicles in critical areas. At the same time, technologies such as facial recognition combined with A.I. convert a large amount of data into private data (such as biometrics data and identity data), thereby posing potential threats to the subjects associated with the data.

In addition, data is highly correlated, meaning it may trigger a domino effect. Applications in many scenarios in the era of big data are highly dependent on data-related operations. While creating more value, big data also dramatically increases the difficulty of managing private data. Compared with the past, the data division under the traditional analysis framework is more pronounced, but it also limits the personal data to a specific scope and department.

In the era of big data, more data are connected and used throughout, and various types of data associated with private data are likely to become highly sensitive. Though technologies such as desensitization and de-identification can be applied to deal with the application process, there are more potential threat points of privacy leakage due to the numerous overall links. The advancement of science and technology has developed our data's accuracy and real-time nature by leaps and bounds. While meeting the needs of production, life, and management, various applications built on such improvements will penetrate more into crucial areas related to the national economy and people's livelihood (such as medical care, health, and finance). Once private data is leaked, there will be terrible consequences.

In addition to the decrease in private data density, the increase in the number, and the high correlation of data, the data in the era of big data also have the feature of strong professional processing. With the rapid development of A.I., new technologies such as deep neural networks have been more widely used. Many AI-based data processing adopts the black-box model, making it difficult for non-professionals to understand the data processing process and quickly leads to ethical issues such as data discrimination and algorithm discrimination.

We are recorded, expressed, simulated, processed, and predicted by the data, intensifying the real space discrimination. Data discrimination is institutionalized and systematized from job and consumption to judicial bias like never before. The algorithm black box shows the imbalance between user data rights and institutional data rights. Data belongs to users, but algorithms belong to institutions; data collection and use are passive for consumers but active for institutions; The algorithm designed by an organization is a model of its will. The algorithm gives the organization excellent data power so that the initiative is always in the hands of the organization.

For institutions, data are transparent. Where there are data, there is an institution. The data belongs to the user, but the user does not know how their information is stored and used. The asymmetry of individual and institutional data rights and the strong professionalism of data processing inevitably lead to the loss of personal privacy boundaries.

The roots of humanity in the privacy paradox

The technical drawbacks that rise with the new features of privacy in the era of big data urgently require the protection of data laws and the evasion of privacy violations, and technology must first come from people and human nature. In the era of big data, we are disgusted by a privacy leak. Still, we cannot reject the convenience brought by technology, so we have indulged in this trend, and eventually, the privacy paradox came into being.

In the era of big data, privacy does not only refer to information deliberately hidden from the public but more to the fact that individuals can decide which information can be disclosed and to whom. At present, the privacy we want to protect most of the time is not scandalous but mundane and commonplace matters. In the Internet Age 2.0, personal information privacy, communication privacy, and space privacy are exposed on the Internet's front or back end. The development of the IoT has exposed people's physiological information and data to the back without reservation end of the Internet. When there is the Internet of Everything, all objects can have sensing functions and media properties, making the physiological information that was never widely spread before becoming an integral part of the spread.

When we become "data-transparent" in the network environment, all personal information is stored in the network's back end. During the COVID-19 pandemic, the nationwide promotion of health codes in China enabled individuals to carry their digital information labels. It becomes our digital twin in a sense. This also raises the question of private ownership: does privacy belong to the individual or the data company that collects the information? In such a media environment, even if users can delete front-end data, their information footprints will become digital footprints and data shadows and be permanently stored and used in the information back end. The Panopticon (an all-seeing prison that Jeremy Bentham proposed in the 19th century) that Michel Foucault predicted seems to have arrived.

Physiological information that is difficult to disguise can undoubtedly reflect the user's status and needs more intuitively than other feedback. When the platform grasps the user's physiological response, intelligent information push and precise advertising become easy. Driven by economic interests, users' physiological information is easily used for various commercial purposes. Through cross-analysis with other information, the commercialized platform will paint a highly accurate portrait of users, which may lead to the recovery of the audience commodity thesis and the reproduction of the magic bullet theory communication effect.

Based on this, the privacy paradox in the era of big data is that though users are more concerned about privacy issues, this attitude does not affect their privacy disclosure behavior, separating their attitude and behavior. However, there is a clear difference between the privacy paradox in social media and the privacy paradox in the IoT. Sharing personal private information on social media is more based on the needs of presence, self-shaping, and social performance. It is an active use of the medium. The initiative to use and refuse privacy leakage is in the hands of users, and resisting the violation of personal privacy will not have a fundamental impact on personal life.

But with the advent of the IoT, as the interaction of private information is the basis for the construction of the IoT, refusing to output personal information means giving up the convenience brought by new technologies, which will form a kind of hypothetical relationship where if one doesn't, one can't. In this media environment, users either give up personal privacy or reject the convenience brought by technology, which gives rise to a new privacy paradox that one cannot have both.

Presently, we obtain user privacy mainly via informed consent. Still, participatory consent is the development direction of future big data behavior, and the ubiquitous pan-media puts users in a state where they must consent. If they don't, they can only not participate in the privacy policy, just like an application on a mobile phone that cannot open if specific access is denied. This is contrary to the ubiquitous use of media, and it is almost impossible to rely on non-participation to deny privacy leakage in the media age.

Is it possible that we say no to convenience? I'm afraid it will be difficult. Based on impact bias, users underestimate the risks associated with things they like and overestimate the risks of things they dislike. For the IoT, which brings convenience to life, people are more likely to adopt an attitude of surrender when privacy is leaked.

No privacy in this era

In March 2018, the Facebook data scandal broke out, shocking the world. The personal data of 87 million Facebook users was sold to a company called Cambridge Analytica L.L.C., which manipulated the data and ultimately managed to influence the voting in the U.K. and the U.S., which then led to Brexit and Trump becoming president.

In January 2019, the scandal was made into the documentary *The Great Hack*, which premiered at the Sundance Film Festival. The film clearly proposes that personal data be a personal asset. It points out that the most influential companies in the world today are tech companies because they hold user data, which is worth more than oil, so tech companies have become the richest.

Cambridge Analytica L.L.C.'s potential users came from a psychological test app on Facebook, which made a psychological portrait of a person by analyzing social behaviors such as liking. "Every American has 5,000 information points. Based on these information points, performing a psychological analysis is enough to construct a person's personality model." When your ten likes are analyzed, the algorithm can know your personality more accurately than your colleagues. It only takes 68 "likes" to estimate a user's skin color (95% accurate), sexual orientation (88% accurate), and political party affiliation

(Republican or Democrat, 85% accurate); with 150 likes data, the algorithm knows more about you than your parents. With over 300 likes, it knows more about you than your spouse; moreover, because everyone has many social friends, the algorithm doesn't need to look directly at your personal information as long as it has access to your friends'.

That is to say: even if you don't use an app yourself, as long as your friends use it, your data will be captured, input into the model, and analyzed by the algorithm. This way, Cambridge Analytica L.L.C. expanded from 270,000 user portraits to 50 million. And the company claimed that based on the 50 million samples, they could accurately predict the behavior of all Americans.

It is reported that China is expected to become the world's largest data producer in 2025. In May 2019, a report released by the Cyberspace Administration of China showed that the scale of the Chinese digital economy in 2018 had reached RMB 31.3 trillion, accounting for 34.8% of its G.D.P. Today, more than 1/3 of our primary economic activity is digital. In addition to individuals, the entire society is becoming increasingly digitalized. Commonly used devices include electronic probes, face recognition, in-vehicle devices, etc.

Meanwhile, data leakage incidents keep happening in China. In April 2018, a food delivery platform was exposed when it leaked user information at a price lower than RMB 0.1 for each piece, including what food was ordered and where. In August 2018, a courier service company was found to have leaked 300 million details of user data for two Bitcoins on a dark web forum, including the senders' names, recipients' names, addresses, phone numbers, and other personal information. In September 2018, a hotel group was reported to be selling its customer data on the dark web. The leaked data included 123 million pieces of official website user registration data, 130 million pieces of traveler identity information, and 240 million detailed room booking records, totaling about 500 million pieces of information. And it was sold for about RMB 370,000. A survey report by the China Consumers Association shows that 85.2% of app users in China have experienced data breaches.

From mobile payments and facial recognition to location sharing, we also pay a huge price for privacy when we enjoy these conveniences. In the first half of 2019, the number of Internet data breaches surged to more than 3,800, reaching an all-time high. Eight hundred seventy million pieces of personal information were sold on the dark web, 773 million email addresses and passwords were stolen, and 590 million Chinese resumes were leaked. The names and phone numbers were disclosed, and the ID numbers, household registrations, marital status, home addresses, etc.

It costs RMB 0.01 to get a piece of personal data and RMB 39 to hack into one's personal information. When a scam call comes in, the con man seems to know more about your resume than yourself. Personal privacy is clearly priced, and we have been sold out without knowing it. There is such a scene in the movie *Eagle Eye*. Two characters are talking in the house, and their sound waves cause the water in a water glass to ripple, which was transcribed into voice information, so the conversation between them was heard. Maybe such an exaggerated plot will hardly happen in real life, but with the development of technology, the violation of privacy is unavoidable. Perhaps such exaggeration might come true.

This is the era of the most privacy and also the era of the least privacy. The big data privacy war is a war that requires joint human action. From individuals to society, we all need to establish privacy awareness and protection mechanisms. How to supervise and achieve a balanced relationship between surveillance and privacy will be a problem that society will have to face and solve for a long time.

Civilization always develops in a spiral, and the progress of an era is bound to be accompanied by various crises and pains. Big data seems to have brought an end to privacy, which we use as a currency to exchange the convenience of life, but the frequent privacy crises in society always alarm us. What should we do ourselves, what should the society do, and what should the state do? The privacy war has only just begun. With the continuous advancement of digitization, by 2035, almost all developed economies will have used big data to construct digital people in the physical society, and the possibility of crime can be judged in advance from digital predictions. Citizens' right to privacy will become the focus of protest and debate in a democratic society. Whenever the government wants, it can get all citizens' information through big data at any time. Humanity will officially enter the era of transparency after 2035.

6.4 Towards Gender Equality

With the enrichment of women's social roles and the simultaneous improvement of consumption power and cognitive ability, the rise of the "she economy" has become an irreversible economic trend for the future. An increasingly open and equal education enables women to continuously escape the job competency trap caused by gender and become the main force of the future economy and consumption. When women have more wealth at their disposal, women show more of their personality, experience, knowledge, and opinions about the present in the Internet age, which will bring marriage, birth, body anxiety, professional women, and other topics into the space of public discussion.

From gender differences to the gender division of labor

Gender differences as an objective existence do not necessarily lead to gender inequality. Still, when gender differences become the basis for constructing an ethical world, they present different ethical characters and temperaments, thereby making the ethical world richer and more vivid. As an ethical culture, Chinese culture's construction of the ethical world and pursuit of moral harmony has always been based on gender differences. It regards the difference between men and women as the core concept of traditional Chinese ethical norms for both genders.

"Yin and Yang, women and men." The construction of the entire ethical world is based on the natural existence of one man and one woman as the starting point. It carries out cultural design and ethical guidance for men and women based on the philosophical concept of yin and yang. Certainly, this kind of cultural design and ethical guidance respects the natural differences between men and women and pursues the ultimate goal of achieving harmonious human relations.

Therefore, based on the original significance of the relationship between both sexes for the ethical world, recognizing and respecting gender differences and establishing ethical identity in gender differences have become unique ethics for human beings and are the "foundations" in the development of human spiritual civilization.

At the same time, it is precisely because of the biological differences because of the gender differences that there is a different division of labor in a family, which in turn produces the division of labor in the public and private fields based on biological gender and the segregation of the labor market based on social gender. This will continue to widen and deepen inequality between men and women.

In 1846, Marx and Engels pointed out that the original division of labor is the division of labor between men and women for the purpose of bearing children. Private ownership is also an inequality caused by the division of labor because of childbirth. It is the root cause of gender inequality. Specifically, in primitive society, the productivity was low, people's divisions of labor were in a natural state, and there was no surplus value, so there was no exploitation. The two genders divided labor based on their physical and living needs. Men hunted and fished, while women collected fruit and handled housework. The two types of labor depended on each other, and men and women managed their own tasks.

With the emergence of monogamous individual families, human beings entered a society based on private ownership. Family economic theorists believe that, as a production unit, everyone in the family has a comparative advantage and establishes their own division of labor in the family according to their comparative advantage.

The gender division of labor within the family burdened women with more responsibility for family care and housework, thus excluded from the public production of society. Housework (including childbirth) became a private matter and lost its public nature.

As a result, men controlled social production, and material production became the leading indicator of social development. Human production has been squeezed out of the public sphere of the social output, and childbirth has become a family affair in the private sphere, a matter exclusive to women. The exclusion of women from the public sphere and the confinement to household chores justifies gender inequality. Under the interaction of patriarchal and capitalist systems, the gender division of labor finally caused gender inequality.

Not a zero-sum game between men and women

For a long time, the existing human spiritual civilization, based on the needs of a male-dominated society, has led to gender inequality that discriminates against women based on recognizing and exaggerating gender differences. Ethical norms were established on the idea that men are superior to women. From the perspective of primitive Confucianism, gender is not only a social division of labor but embodies the moral judgment that men are superior to women. This ideology confines women to the private sphere, making them an instrument suitable for patriarchal needs.

With the profound changes in modern society, modern means of labor have gradually eliminated strength and gender segregation, and women's ability and value have been greatly released as they participate in social production. The pursuit of gender equality has become one of the significant means of progress in modern society that is different from traditional society. Meanwhile, the need for women to keep pace with social development and work procedures has gradually become prominent.

Women have gone from being a ruled and oppressed class to now having the right to be able to participate in social production independently. They have gone through a hard journey from their initial demands for an independent personality and the right to live to their political demands for equality between men and women. However, the biological differences between genders make women still bear the inescapable biological responsibility of childbirth. The confinement of traditional ideas also makes women take a larger share of family work, thus creating an unavoidable contradiction with the continuous individual needs of society.

On the one hand, with the social voice and institutional efforts for modern Chinese women's liberation and equality between men and women, women's social status, economic status, and social responsibility have unprecedentedly improved. Since the reform and opening-up period, many professional women have emerged in China's transition from an agricultural society to an industrial society, where they have made great contributions to promoting social development and creating social wealth.

However, due to the traditional ethical expectations of women's family roles and their physiological reasons, in addition to men's roles in the family and their corresponding moral obligations, women's status has not been redefined or institutionally guaranteed with the development of modern society. This makes traditional ethics enter a vacuum period under the impact of modernization, which leads women to face a new ethical dilemma: a fierce conflict between the dual ethical identities of women's family roles and social roles.

On the other hand, under the social wave of pursuing freedom, general equality, and calling for gender equality, coupled with the boost of industrialization and information development to the transformation of human production modes and lifestyles, the gender differences that were taken for granted in traditional human spiritual civilization are increasingly blurred and even chaotic in the modern society, which eventually leads to the ethical alienation of gender differences.

As a result, an over-interpretation of gender equality has weakened the concept of gender equality or eliminated the differences in ethical characteristics between men and women, so gender equality is misunderstood as meaning that men and women are the same. And this misunderstanding will inevitably lead to the ambiguity of the ethical obligations of women and men based on different ethical personalities and moral temperaments, which in turn breeds new inequalities.

Obviously, gender differences are often complementary differences between the two sexes. That is, each sex exists with its different conditions, characteristics, and expertise and needs to be the objectivity of the other. It is like the two sides of a coin are inseparable, but each has its own status and value. The progress of social history is the two sexes progressing hand in hand with mutual dependence and support, during which the values created by men for men and women for women are shown.

Today, human spiritual civilization's cultural interpretation of gender differences has already transcended the natural physiological differences between men and women. In the ethical world, men and women have irreplaceable ethical characters and moral temperaments.

Under the impact of modernization, gender issues will last for a long time, and there may be more deconstruction and construction of gender ethics in the future. However, whether it is an emotional outburst or a calm and serious discussion, among the various opinions, the only certainty is that the real gender equality should be that women and men have the same dignity, rather than seeking to be absolutely the same externally.

With maliciousness and labels stripped, we will find that many contradictions are not gender contradictions, and the relationship between men and women has never been a zero-sum game. It is foreseeable that by around 2035, human society, at least in some advanced economies, will no longer be gender-differentiated. The equality between men and women will change from relative parity in the past to absolute equality.

6.5 The Ups and Downs of Scientific Research During the COVID-19 Pandemic

The year 2020 will be remembered in history because of the COVID-19 pandemic. The pandemic has become the most critical variable affecting the global economy and international politics. It has exacerbated social uncertainty so that different problems continue to emerge in various fields. Education, medical care, and even social ideology are under severe scrutiny.

Also, the pandemic, like a medical event, has triggered the most significant turning point in the history of modern science. In the fall of 2019, scientists did little research on the coronavirus because it had never existed.

As of June 5, 2022, the pandemic has spread to 228 countries and territories, infecting more than 525 million people and killing more than 6.3 million people. This sparked unprecedented efforts in the scientific community, dramatically shifting the focus of scientific research.

Certainly, the pandemic has also exposed many problems in scientific research. For example, the vicious competition in academia forces researchers to use the pandemic as a chance to pursue fame and fortune. Identifying and encouraging beneficial research and eliminating impetuousness and utilitarianism will be essential issues for scientific research in the post-COVID era.

Unprecedented scientific efforts

The pandemic has unexpectedly shattered the once linear, smooth, and predictable society. For scientific research, it has shifted the focus of scientific research, accelerated the sharing of scientific information, and brought the findings of infectious disease research to the public attention and popularized them.

First, thousands of researchers temporarily set aside previously consuming research topics during the pandemic and began studying the pandemic instead. In just a few months, there formed the trend where scientific research became focused on COVID-19.

According to PubMed (a free search engine accessing the MEDLINE database of references and abstracts on life sciences and biomedical topics primarily), 74,000 COVID-19 papers have been published on PubMed since the beginning of 2020, which was several times the number of documents on polio, measles, cholera, and dengue that have been around for centuries. For Ebola, one of the most aggressive infectious diseases that emerged in 1976, there are only 9,700 papers. As of September 2021, the most authoritative medical journal, *The New England Journal of Medicine* (N.E.J.M.), has received a total of 30,000 submissions in 2021, and more than half are COVID-19 articles.

Like the famous Manhattan Project and the Apollo Space Program, the pandemic has assembled many scientists. The Spanish Flu of 1918, the threat of malaria on the tropical battlefields of World War II, and the rise of polio in the years following the war all triggered major turning points. The Ebola and Zika pandemics have also prompted a temporary surge in funding and publications in recent years. The COVID-19 pandemic is undoubtedly a new turning point that has led to an unprecedented shift in the focus of scientific research.

In a survey of 2,500 U.S., Canada, and Europe researchers, a Harvard research team found that 32% of them had turned their attention to the COVID-19 pandemic.

For example, neuroscientists who study the sense of smell have begun investigating why patients with Covid-19 lose their sense of smell. Michael D. L. Johnson of the University of Arizona usually studies the toxic effects of copper on bacteria. Still, when he learned that the SARS-CoV-2 virus persists for a shorter period of time on copper surfaces than on other materials, he partially turned to the study of the vulnerability of the virus on the metal surface. In fact, for modern medicine, no disease has ever been examined so intensely by so many integrative disciplines in such a short time.

Second, research on the coronavirus is being shared at a surprising speed during the pandemic, which has also transformed science from a slow, closed effort to one that is more flexible and transparent. Traditionally, a study is published through a lengthy process: the paper is first submitted to a journal, which sends it to peers for review; if it passes the peer review (which could take months), after paying an expensive charge, the paper will be published.

Obviously, this system is not suitable for the rapidly spreading COVID-19. Thus, during the COVID -19 pandemic, biomedical scientists can upload preliminary versions or preprints of their papers to freely accessible websites so others can analyze their findings.

Though this practice had slowly become popular before 2020, the pandemic has undoubtedly accelerated its promotion and popularization because this is important for sharing information about COVID-19 and has the potential to become mainstream in modern biomedical studies.

Preprints have accelerated the advancement of science, and the pandemic has accelerated the use of preprints. Earlier in 2021, a repository called medRxiv (med archive) held about 1,000 preprints. By the end of October, over 12,000 people had access to this repository.

In addition, the pandemic has also exposed the threats of infectious diseases that were neglected in the past and made little-known findings of infectious disease research known to the public. About 90 years ago, humans could not observe viruses; in 2020, 10 days after the first case of COVID-19 was detected, Chinese scientists uploaded the viral genome sequence of SARS-CoV-2. As of November 2021, 197,000 viral sequences had been uploaded.

In addition, researchers have begun to uncover how SARS-CoV-2 compares to other coronaviruses (likely hosts) in wild bats; how it invades and combines with our cells; and how the immune system overreacts to it, resulting in COVID-19 symptoms. Arguably, people are learning about this virus faster than any other virus in history.

Pandemic exposes weaknesses in scientific research

The pandemic has assembled unprecedented efforts in the scientific community, demonstrating the inherent logic of the modernization of science and technology. Still, it has also exposed many problems in the scientific community during the pandemic. As a unique disaster, the pandemic has put academia in the face of a significant test.

Biomedical academia is a pyramid. Each biomedical professor nurtures an average of six doctoral students during their career, but only 16% of students receive tenure. Thus, the pandemic has provided an excellent opportunity for many researchers to make a splash: amid a major outbreak where everyone is affected and desperate for information, any new paper can immediately attract the attention of the international media and possibly be cited extensively.

Governments, charities, and universities allocate vast sums of money to Covid-19 research. In March 2020, the U.S. Congress gave the U.S. National Science Foundation additional special funding of US$ 75 million for COVID-19 research. These factors have attracted an influx of scientists into the field of COVID-19 studies and encouraged a deluge of sloppy, utilitarian, and hyped research at the expense of academic rigor.

The chances of the pandemic also fall unfairly on the scientific community. Among scientists, as in other fields, women do more childcare, housework, and teaching than men and are more requested by students for emotional support. As the pandemic spreads, female scientists are increasingly burdened, unable to devote more time to understanding new research areas or starting an entirely new research project. Research from Santa Clara University shows that women spend 9% less research time than men due to the stress of COVID-19.

Compared to 2019, the proportion of papers with women as first authors in the medRxiv preprint repository has dropped by nearly 44%. Compared with papers from the same journals in 2021, 19% fewer women were first authors of published COVID-19 papers, while men led over 80% of national COVID-19 research teams in 87 countries. Male scientists are cited four times as often as female scientists in U.S. news coverage of the pandemic.

Scientists of color in the U.S. have also suffered a more challenging time navigating than their white peers because of unique challenges that consume their time and energy. Black, Latino, and Indigenous scientists are most at risk of losing a loved one, which adds mourning to their list of duties.

Science suffers from the so-called Matthew effect, where small successes snowball toward larger advantages, regardless of merit. Also, early hurdles remain. Young researchers who are too busy caring for or grieving for others to change their views may suffer lasting consequences from a year of low productivity.

The COVID-19 pandemic has greatly changed scientific research, including a shift in the focus of scientific research and accelerated sharing of scientific information. Meanwhile, the concerted efforts of scientists worldwide to respond to the outbreak have brought invaluable experience in dealing with other global infectious disease threats in the future.

The pandemic has also exposed the weaknesses of scientific research, such as distorted incentives, wasteful practices, inequality, biomedical bias, etc. How to identify and encourage beneficial research and eliminate impetuousness and utilitarianism will be an important issue for scientific research in the post-COVID era.

6.6 Social Development Requires Urgent Correction and Updates

Looking back at the evolution of human civilization, the entire society has always shown a strong correspondence between the two "schedules" of technological genealogy and cultural context. Every leap of science and technology once again provides opportunities for cultural prosperity. From papermaking to printing, the dissemination of human knowledge has achieved a qualitative breakthrough, and orders of magnitude have improved the popularization of public knowledge. In the mid-1760s, replacing manual tools with machine tools in England was a profound change in the history of technology and a great leap in cultural transformation, including the concept of family, marriage, and blood kinship. While promoting the transformation of social relations, such a replacement also triggered a great leap in cultural transformation, including the change of family, marriage, and kinship concepts, as well as the development of society from compulsory restraint to democratization.

Though the integration of technology and culture is creating more possibilities in the digital age, the changes from science and technology to culture are not only reflected in the links of production and dissemination. The rise of the platform-based ecosystem has reshaped the value chain composition and organization of the cultural industry and also altered its original structure. New business forms and models continue to emerge, and culture and related industries are integrated and coexist, becoming a new force for economic growth while updating people's understanding and opinions on cultural content. But thriving science and technology, while reshaping society, has also pushed human ethics into an unprecedented no-man's-land.

In every sense, we are in a downward age. Regardless of politics, economics, or culture, all standards are aligned with the lowest, and all low-level standards have become new standards. When honor is discarded, gentility is gone, shamelessness is advocated, under the one-sided and one-size-fits-all thinking mode of national utilitarianism and pragmatism, the system where capital seeks profit is rampant. In such an era, there is an urgent need for humanistic thought to guide and help people's spiritual lives.

The human values system faces challenges

As technology continues to advance, people have entered the age of electricity, from the age of steam to the age of atoms and information. However, while technology enriches the material world where people live, it also makes people face more and more crises of cognition, survival, and belief.

In the 21st century, under the influence of the rapid advancement of science and technology, human society's structure and spiritual outlook keep undergoing dramatic changes. Communication technology, the Internet, big data, cloud computing, blockchain, A.I., genetic engineering, and virtual technology have integrated information and entities into a data-driven economy. The intelligent networking of the entire society is causing a profound revolution in production mode, lifestyle, thinking patterns, and governance.

However, though emerging technologies have ushered in the dawn of the Fourth Industrial Revolution, it has also made some people (rational) conceited again. In real life, rationality degenerates into algorithms and calculations, and calculations degenerate into plotting. While the new technological and industrial revolutions are vigorously promoting social development, there are additional environmental, ecological, and ethical risks and problems such as personal spiritual loss, absence of beliefs, and a crisis of meaning. These are all in urgent need of values remodeling through humanistic spiritual guidance.

Global warming haunts many people. In 2020, a team of 93 scientists published a paleoclimate data record spanning the past 12,000 years, including 1,319 data records. The data comes from samples, such as lake sediment, marine sediment, peat, cave sediment, coral, and glacial ice cores, collected from 679 locations worldwide.

As a result, the researchers could map changes in surface air temperature over the past 12,000 years and then compare it to century-average temperatures between 1800 and 1900 to track changes that the Industrial Revolution may have triggered. As expected, temperatures were much lower at the start of the 12,000-year-period than the 19th-century baseline. But over the next few thousand years, temperatures rose steadily, surpassing the baseline at last.

Temperatures peaked 6,500 years ago, and the earth has been slowly cooling down ever since. The cooling rate after the peak was minor, only about 0.1°C per 1,000 years. However, human activity has raised the average temperature by as high as 1°C since the mid-19th century. This is an astonishing peak in a relatively short period of time, rising even higher than the peak 6,500 years ago.

Climate change has shattered the balance of light and heat irradiated by the sun to the earth and their reflection. And the most direct consequence of the broken balance is exacerbated climate disasters. The nonprofit organization Germanwatch published a report in 2020 that analyzes extreme climates, including storms, floods, and heat, but excluded slowly occurring environmental changes such as the rising sea level, warming oceans, and melting glaciers. The report shows that between 2000 and 2019, about 11,000 extreme meteorological calamities broke out worldwide.

The infection problem that we once thought to have been controlled is back. Climate changes have partly caused the geographic expansion of ticks and tick-borne pathogens. The possibility of transmitting tick-borne and other infections is further increased due to the lack of global governance, policies, and international cooperation to mitigate climate changes and promote a more balanced relationship between humans and nature. In addition, since the mid-20th century, the surface temperature of the Arctic has continued to rise, nearly doubling the rate of warming compared to the global average. Rising temperatures are melting sea ice, snow cover, and permafrost, threatening the lives of about seven million people. For example, permafrost stores mercury and other persistent environmental pollutants and infectious agents, and once thawed, these substances are released and pose health risks.

The abuse of antibiotics, combined with natural evolution, has created increasingly dangerous microbes. According to the U.S. Centers for Disease Control and Prevention, there are over 2.8 million cases of antibiotic resistance in the U.S. alone each year, killing more than 35,000 people. In India, neonatal infections caused by antibiotic resistance kill nearly 60,000 newborn babies yearly. The U.N. fears that by 2050, 10 million people worldwide will die each year from drug-resistant infections.

Antibiotic resistance not only seriously harms human health but also inflicts huge burdens and losses on the economy. The U.S. medical system alone needs to spend US$ 20 billion to solve the problem of drug resistance every year. British economist Jim O'Neill estimates that by 2050, global antibiotic resistance will have caused a cumulative economic loss of US$ 100 trillion. In addition, the reports of the World Bank and the Food and Agriculture Organization of the U.N. also pointed out that if the problem of antibiotic resistance is not solved by 2050, the global annual G.D.P. will have declined by 1.1% to 3.8%, which is as terrible as the 2008 financial crisis.

Computerization is revolutionizing new areas of work and recreation all the time. Still, it also comes at a cost, including rising unemployment, a widening digital divide, a breakdown in how traditional communities are formed and maintained, and the inability (now, perhaps ever) of online interactions to replace traditional communities fully, etc. The social structure leans towards globalization, and various regional cultures are blended in multiple forms. A.I. is developed, and there are robust systems that rule the lives of all people by various means.

In the present highly developed mobile Internet, social media with labels everywhere outlines a bizarre world based on algorithms; male and female anchors with a broken reputation apply technology to create a simulacrum that erodes reality; all information, knowledge, and opinions are easily obtainable, and the massive amount of information, like randomly coded symbols, piles up the ruins of data, indicating our separation from others in this era.

The rate at which the legal and aesthetic systems are constructed does not follow the anxiety towards the rapid advancement of technology, which scares the public. Both the Confucian benevolence, righteousness, and etiquette that Chinese traditional culture has complied with for thousands of years and the democratic system of Western liberalism have been gradually shattered with the advent of the Internet. Therefore, at the juncture of the age of machines, people are confused and hesitant about what remains unknown in this age in the face of this huge vacuum period.

When rewriting the world, human lifestyle, and inherent values, the ever-advancing technology has also taken human beings to an unprecedented no-man's land. It is not until this very moment that people more deeply note and feel that the religions, humanistic thoughts, and values that have guided mankind in the past can no longer cope with the changes brought about by science and technology to a certain extent. In other words, human beings' current thinking and interpretation of religions and humanities can no longer guide them to deal with the current no-man's land and the future road to no-man's land.

Meanwhile, the increasing prosperity of pragmatism in modern business society has weakened the humanistic spirit. As the era of the knowledge economy arrives, the added value of knowledge attached to items will obviously increase the items' value. Therefore, in a knowledge society, knowledge can survive only in application. Moreover, since World War II, natural science has occupied the top position in leading social development through the information revolution and new technological revolution, and technological civilization has dominated the contemporary world. Compared with the natural sciences, the development of the humanities appears weak.

When peace and development have become the theme of the times, the humanities and social sciences cannot directly create economic value in a short time nor be a vital force in promoting world economic growth and technological progress. However, as the humanities abandoned itself in the past and failed to respond keenly to modernity, it cannot provide effective conceptual guidance and help promptly solve complex problems in the new situation.

From the perspective of specific higher education practice, the humanities and social sciences seem to be gradually becoming marginalized: in a school planning outline called *Profile 2016* published by the University of Amsterdam in 2014, funding was planned to be cut, and some linguistic majors canceled. Also, it was designed that the remaining majors of the other humanities in colleges, including philosophy, history, Dutch literature, and so on, be merged into a humanities degree, and the school's focus is placed on more career-oriented majors. U.S. appropriations to the humanities also fell from US$ 400 million (by 2016 U.S. dollars) in 1979 to US$ 150 million (by 2016 U.S. dollars) in 2015. This is a time when crises and new opportunities coexist, and industrial civilization's development urgently needs the humanities' guidance and correction.

Science and technology ethics towards renewal

The integration of technology and culture and their development to a new height organically combine elements such as cultural content, ideas, and forms with the spirit, methods, and theories of science and technology, to change the value and quality of products and create new content, forms, functions, and services. This embodies a process of innovation and renews the social order.

Robert King Merton, a representative figure of American structural functionalism, placed technology on the visual threshold of social change and explored the influence of culture and technology on society. Merton believes that it is the lack of the conceptual framework required by the sociocultural structure of the technology itself that hinders the advancement of technology because, no matter how the surrounding culture affects the development of scientific knowledge, no matter how science and technology ultimately change the society, the effects come from the changing institutional and organizational structure of technology.

Though the humanities cannot replace the government and the public to formulate public policies nor deprive the people and elected officials of their decision-making power, it can provide the public with information so that the public make informed decisions based on helpful information, which is also the basis for the survival of the future industrial world.

In the early 1970s, then-U.S. President Richard M. Nixon initiated the R&D of supersonic transport. At that time, Nixon wanted to make a significant technical achievement like President John F. Kennedy's Apollo space program, and he chose the supersonic transport plane, the government-funded cooperation with Boeing and other aircraft companies to develop supersonic aircraft for civil aviation or bombers.

Dr. Melvin Calvin (a biochemist and Nobel Prize for Chemistry winner), as a member of the Science Advisory Board, led a government advisory group to investigate this plan. They advised the president that, considering the economic benefits and environmental impacts, such as loud acoustic shocks and extremely high-altitude air pollution, the supersonic transport plan would lead to more loss than gain. During the dispute, Dr. Calvin decided to testify publicly in Congress against the supersonic transport program, and consequently, the program was denied by Congress.

At the Congressional hearing, Dr. Calvin and other scientists pointed out that technical decision-making should not be limited to rational technical considerations in a narrow sense but extend rationality and objective thinking to the technical level, to the broader society, economic and political aspects. In other words, ethics, sociology, and even historical and philosophical studies must be able to keep up with the times at the level of social decision-making. Should the advancement of science and technology receive no support from the humanities, there will be inevitable harm to all mankind.

In the social context of technology and culture, technology is a social, organizational system that is slowly forming and changing. Obviously, technology benefits the economy of the whole society and transforms the culture, and renews the social order, which is visible in the industrial revolution. This means that the pan-industrial revolution represented by information technologies such as A.I. and big data will reshape a new and ready-to-go social order, which must contain new and old values and society-valued ideas that are successfully combined.

Inspired by the triple helix of genes, the innovation triple helix theory creatively proposes a new paradigm of innovation. It believes that the innovation support system must build a helical connection mode, and this entwined helix is composed of three forces: the administrative chain composed of local or regional governments and their subordinate institutions, the production chain composed of vertically and horizontally connected companies, and the techno-scientific chain composed of research and academic institutions. In addition to performing the functions of knowledge creation, wealth production, and policy coordination, the three forces also derive new functions through mutual interaction and eventually breed innovation based on knowledge reproduction.

Technology, culture, and social order are in line with the innovation triple helix theory and grow and develop based on it. Among them, social order is the goal of cultural pursuit and scientific and technological exploration. Still, its explanatory significance is neither in culture nor can it be confined to science and technology. Social order is an independent and substantial spiral.

The triple helix of culture, science, technology, and social order work together and promote innovation, forming a mutually causal relationship. They are the formed core attraction of the system, enabling the innovation triple helix to come into being. The establishment of social order and the dissemination of the dominant culture and scientific and technological progress promote the upward spiral of innovation and become the internal driving force for the establishment of the innovation triple helix.

On the one hand, the economic attributes of technological creation determine that the technology must be tightly connected with the external market. Meanwhile, the uncertainty of the external market reacts to the cultural, technological, and social order. It requires culture to guide the path. And it truly promotes healthy social development through the mutual promotion of culture, technology, and social order.

On the other hand, the primary driving force for the formation of culture, technology, and social order comes from the respective needs of the three parties. The innovation of cultural activation requires the support of science and technology and the guidance of values; the social order reflects the new ideas of the times and needs the embodiment of cultural content and the support of science and technology; the leap-forward development of scientific and technological milestones is inseparable from the overall cultivation of a social and cultural atmosphere and the guidance of a new social order.

The progress of human society, on the surface, is one technological invention after another that promotes social progress; from a mid-scope perspective, it is technological innovation that brings cultural innovation and new modes of survival and lifestyles to human society; from a deep perspective, it is the integration and innovation of technology and culture that creates a new human spiritual group and breeds a new social value system.

Obviously, the growth of human civilization is by no means the growth of external material but the establishment of inner spirit, which is an upgrade from the spread of individual spiritual self-discipline to the overall social order. When the role of science and technology in the industrial society gradually becomes more robust and undergoes a transformation from the technical level to the driving force of the commercial economy, how to truly integrate technology and culture to become an essential support for social development and civilization progress is an inevitable topic of the times. Looking to the future, with the reconstruction of the technological society and the resetting of thinking patterns, the world will change, and there will be completely new meanings.

In the post-COVID-19 era, human society will enter a new period of coexisting with crises as the world patterns have undergone irreversible changes due to the impact of the pandemic. In the name of scientific and technological progress, humans have destroyed the environment at an unprecedented level and entered a no-man's land in exploring science and technology, science and life. When it is at its limit, the earth will heal itself in its own unique way. In the prehistoric age of dinosaurs, dinosaurs ruled the earth. When their reproduction posed a significant threat to the planet's ecology, the earth reorganized the entire ecosystem through volcanic eruptions. Perhaps, the present COVID-19 pandemic is a warning from the earth to mankind. Suppose humanity fails to respect nature and protect the environment but continues to recklessly use the advancement of science and technology to destroy the ecological balance indefinitely. In that case, it is foreseeable that the next catastrophe of mankind will be more deadly than the coronavirus. In the face of this virus test, human society has failed. It engages in international confrontation for various political purposes rather than uniting. Predicting how selfish humans will ultimately take nature's warnings and lessons is difficult. Perhaps, the next crisis will break out around 2035.

References

Beijing Science and Technology Development Exchange Center. *African New Economy White Paper* 2019.

CAICT China Academy of Information and Communications Technology. *Global Artificial Intelligence Strategy and Policy Observation.*

Caitong Securities. *Report on Online Medical Care: Technology Helps Fight the Pandemic, Best Time for Online Medical Care.* 2020

Deloitte Touche Tohmatsu Limited. *White Paper on Global Artificial Intelligence Development.*

Huang Guixia. "Inequality Between Men and Women: From the Private Sphere to the Public Sphere—From the Perspective of 'The Origin of Family, Private Ownership and the State.'" *Journal of Shandong Women's University*, no. 4 (2017): 1–8.

Lan, Yun. "Research on the Development Trend of the Sharing Economy in China." *Modern Marketing* 10, late issue (2018): 14.

Li, Chunhui, Hu Bo, Weng Yuhua, and Huang Yuanyu. "The Current Situation and Clinical Research Progress of Gene Therapy." *Life Science Instruments* 17, no. Z1 (2019): 3–12.

Li, Jun, Li Xilin, and Wang Tuo. "Conceptual Connotation, Development Trend and Counter-measures of Digital Trade." *International Trade*, no. 5 (2021): 12–21. DOI:10.14114/j.cnki.itrade.2021.05.003.

Liu, Yuanchun. "Reshaping of Globalization in the Post-Covid Times." *China Clothing*, no. 12 (2020): 9.

Mu, Jie. "Opportunities, Challenges and Prospects of the Central Bank's Implementation of the Legal Digital Currency DCEP." *The Economist*, no. 3 (2020): 95–105. DOI:10.16158/j.cnki.51-1312/f.2020.03.010.

SPDB International. *In-depth Report on the Online Medical Care: the Decisive Moment is Here.* 2020

State Information Center. *China Sharing Economy Development Report* (2021).

Tencent Research Institute. *2020 Tencent Artificial Intelligence White Paper.*

Wei, Chenzi, and Ji Li. "Difficulties and Countermeasures in the Supervision of Human Assisted Reproductive Technology and Surrogacy." *X Soft Health Science* 33, no. 12 (2019): 39–42.

Xiao, Wanjun, and Xian Guoming. "The Development of RCEP: the Game of Interests of All Parties and China's Strategic Choice." *International Economic Cooperation*, no. 2 (2020): 12–25.

Yu Weidong. "The Dilemma and Integration Model of Muslim Immigrants Blending into Western European Countries." *New Silk Road Journal*, no. 2 (2018): 96–108.

Zhang, Hui, and Zhang Yanhua. "The Emergence and Response to the Gap Between the Rich and the Poor in Contemporary China." *Economic Research Guide*, no. 25 (2020): 4–5, 48.

Zhang, Qidi. "Concern about 'Differentiation': Why the U.S. Economy Presents a 'K-shaped' Recovery." *Financial Market Research*, no. 2 (2021): 64–69.

Zhang, Qingmin. "The Covid Pandemic Tests Global Public Health Governance." *Northeast Asia Forum* 29, no. 4 (2020): 43–59, 127. DOI:10.13654/j.cnki.naf.2020.04.004.

Zhang, Xiaheng. "Research on the Development of the Gig Economy." *Reform and Strategy* 36, no. 8 (2020): 46–53. DOI:10.16331/j.cnki.issn1002-736x.2020.08.005.

Zhang, Zunyue, Wang Kunhua, Tang Li, Long Yanxi, and Wang Huawei. "Ethical Thinking on Human Assisted Reproductive Technology." *Medical Contention* 10, no. 6 (2019): 38–41. DOI:10.13276/j.issn.1674-8913.2019.06.010.

Zhongtai Securities. *In-depth Report on the Online Medical Care: Online Medical Care On the Rise.* 2020

Index

ABOUT THE AUTHOR

Kevin Chen is a renowned science and technology writer and scholar. He was a visiting scholar at Columbia University, a postdoctoral scholar at Cambridge, and an invited course professor at Peking University. He has served as a special commentator and columnist for the *People's Daily*, CCTV, the China Business Network, SINA, NetEase, and many other media outlets. He has published monographs in numerous domains, including finance, science and technology, real estate, medical treatments, and industrial design. He currently lives in Hong Kong.